# STAYING YOUNG

# STAYING YOUNG

How to Prevent, Slow
or Reverse More Than
60 Signs of Aging

Tom Monte
and the Editors of

## *PREVENTION*

Magazine

BERKLEY BOOKS, NEW YORK

This book is intended as a reference volume only, not as a medical manual. The information given here is designed to help you make informed decisions about your health. It is not intended as a substitute for any treatment that may have been prescribed by your doctor. If you suspect that you have a medical problem, we urge you to seek competent medical help.

STAYING YOUNG

A Berkley Book / published by arrangement with
Rodale Press, Inc.

PRINTING HISTORY
Rodale Press edition published 1994
Berkley edition / March 1996

All rights reserved.
Copyright © 1994 by Rodale Press, Inc.
*Prevention* is a registered trademark of Rodale Press, Inc.
This book may not be reproduced in whole or in part,
by mimeograph or any other means, without permission.
For information address: Rodale Press, Inc.,
33 E. Minor Street, Emmaus, Pennsylvania 18098.

ISBN: 0-425-15251-0

BERKLEY®
Berkley Books are published by The Berkley Publishing Group,
200 Madison Avenue, New York, New York 10016.
BERKLEY and the "B" design
are trademarks belonging to Berkley Publishing Corporation.

PRINTED IN THE UNITED STATES OF AMERICA

10 9 8 7 6 5 4 3 2

# ACKNOWLEDGMENTS

Special thanks to Maria Fiatarone, M.D., chief of the physiology laboratory at the U.S. Department of Agriculture's Human Nutrition Research Center on Aging at Tufts University in Boston and assistant professor in the division on aging at Harvard Medical School, for reviewing the manuscript of this book and offering valuable advice. Also thanks to Christine Dreisbach, senior research associate at Rodale Press, for her meticulous attention to research, fact checking and shepherding of the manuscript through the review process.

# CONTENTS

# PART II: LOOKING GREAT

# PART III: THINKING AND FEELING YOUNG

# INTRODUCTION

## A New Definition of Aging

**To** many of us, that first gray hair or faint line in the brow comes as a shock. Somehow, we never thought *we* would get old. With the unconsciously vain optimism of youth, we thought we'd stay young forever.

No one can halt the hands of time. But we *can* halt much of the deterioration—both mental and physical—that we have routinely associated with aging. "Many of the things we blame on aging really have nothing to do with getting older," says Ben Douglas, Ph.D., author of *AgeLess: Living Younger Longer* and professor of anatomy at the University of Mississippi Medical Center in Jackson.

More and more evidence suggests that how we approach aging can make all the difference in how the years affect us. People slow down as they grow older because they *expect* to, says Deepak Chopra, M.D., in his book *Ageless Body, Timeless Mind.* We think of older people as wrinkled and plump, with gnarled hands and feeble gait—and gradually, inexorably, we let ourselves become those people.

But you *can* retain vigor, alertness, muscle tone and a strong immune system in your later years. You can also greatly reduce your chances of experiencing debilitating ailments such as heart disease, osteoporosis, diabetes and cataracts. You can continue to *look* good, too. And you don't need to visit expensive spas or rejuvenation specialists or supply yourself with large bottles of expensive potions and powders. You can accomplish this yourself—with regular trim-down, tune-up exercises accompanied by healthful eating, plus styling tricks and skin-care techniques that put the brakes on what we incorrectly assume are inevitable signs of aging.

This book tells you how, step-by-step. In Part I, "Feeling Good," you'll find tips from experts to help prevent and cope with ailments ranging from angina to vision problems. One important strategy is maintaining your fitness: "Use it or lose it" may be a cliché, but it's true. "A lot of the effects of aging are self-inflicted," says Terence Kavanagh, M.D., director of the Toronto Rehabilitation Center in Ontario. "The less you do, the easier you fatigue. And the more you fatigue, the less you are able to do."

There's plenty of evidence that exercise improves not only your ability to get around, work harder and play harder but also your mood, resistance to infections, reaction time, sex life and mental abilities. And it's never too late to start. You can "turn back the clock" whether you're 32 or 82. No matter what condition you're in now, a reasonable exercise program can restore fitness, build strength, improve aerobic capacity, tone your muscles and help keep you at your ideal weight. "By taking yourself from a sedentary state to a physically trained state, you can, in effect, reduce your biological age by 10 or 20 years," says Roy Shepard, M.D., Ph.D., a professor of applied physiology at the University of Toronto.

And we're not talking running marathons or working out with massive weights for hours a day. Look at the 756 athletes, ages 35 to 94, who participated in events such as rowing, swimming and track and field in the 1985 World Masters Games. "We found some people in their late 60s and 70s who had about the same cardiopulmonary fitness as you would expect from sedentary 25-year-olds," says Dr. Kavanagh. And most of them trained less than seven hours a week in preparation for the games. "These weren't fanatical trainers in any sense. It seems that even moderate exercise can push aging back," he says.

But physical activity is only part of the prescription for staying young. What we eat—and don't eat—makes an enormous difference in how we age. The right foods can help protect against ailments such as heart disease, cancer, osteoporosis, stroke, gastrointestinal problems, arthritis and high blood pressure. In these pages, you'll read about exciting new research on antioxidants—substances in foods that neutralize harmful free radicals within our bodies—which apparently have incredibly far-reaching effects on aging. And how getting enough of certain nutrients can increase resistance to infectious diseases. And so on.

Our appearance can also affect how we age. Most of us know that when we look good, we feel good—with that extra bounce in our step and sparkle in our eye. In Part II, "Looking Great," you'll get the latest advice on keeping your skin, hair, nails and teeth looking their best.

And, finally, mental fitness is as critical to staying young as physical fitness. Attitude, for example, is an important ingredient in how long you live—and how *well* you live. Studies suggest that a dour outlook may worsen your health, says William Rakowski, Ph.D., from the Center for Gerontology and Health Care Research at Brown University in Providence. In Part III, "Thinking and Feeling Young," experts tell you how to keep your wits sharp, conquer depression and deal with worry, loneliness and stress.

No one can live forever. But you *can* take action to help yourself feel and look your best throughout your life, and that's what this book is about. Picking it up is the first step to discovering a whole new definition of *aging*.

Tom Monte

# PART I
## Feeling Good

# AEROBICS

### Have Fun and Delay Aging

**Many** of us avoid exercise because the thought of it conjures up images of pain and sweat. The truth is that a health-restoring exercise program isn't painful at all. Scientists tell us that simple pleasures like regular walks in the park or bicycle rides through your neighborhood will increase your chances of living longer, give you greater vitality and a more youthful appearance and improve your outlook on life.

Going on a brisk stroll with your Great Dane, step climbing to the oldies or piling up the miles on a treadmill while watching TV all provide an aerobic workout. You draw greater quantities of air into your lungs and deliver more oxygen to your heart, brain and muscles—in fact, you oxygenate virtually every cell in your body.

One of the biggest benefits of regular aerobic exercise is that you increase the maximum amount of oxygen your muscles can absorb and utilize, a measurement known as $VO_2$ max. As people age, their $VO_2$ max tends to drop steadily, causing a decline in stamina. The good news is that by stepping up your aerobic activity, you can maintain a higher $VO_2$ max and hold the line against the decline. In short, exercise slows the aging process.

### WHAT EXERCISE CAN DO FOR YOU

Exercise will help you lose weight if you need to, simply because you burn calories that are stored as fat. That alone will improve your self-image, but the psychological benefits don't stop there.

"Exercise increases the heart's stroke volume," says Craig Cisar, Ph.D., a professor of exercise physiology at San Jose State University in California. "That means that your heart is capable of pumping more blood per beat and therefore requires fewer beats to do the same amount of work." Your heart is thus more efficient, both at rest and during exertion. You will be able to perform more work before reaching your maximal heart rate, and your heart will have time to fill properly between beats.

Regular exercise—particularly if it results in weight loss—may also raise your HDLs (high density lipoproteins), the "good" cholesterol. HDLs literally shepherd "bad" cholesterol back to your liver for disposal and thus reduce your chances of suffering a heart attack. In fact, HDLs rise even faster for those who are overweight and begin an exercise program. Scientists believe that the combined benefits of losing weight and working out cause the body to raise its HDL count more rapidly.

Exercise can also help reduce stress. Most people begin an aerobic exercise program to cut down their risk of coronary artery disease or to help lose weight, according to David J. Mersy, M.D., chairman of the department of family medicine at St. Paul–Ramsey Medical Center. But many of these same people stick with exercise even after they attain their goals because of the lift working out gives them: They no longer feel as anxious or depressed. They can handle stress better, and they find they have a sunnier outlook on life.

A study in the *Journal of the American Medical Association* showed that even a little exercise dramatically lowers your risk from dying from heart disease and cancer. The scientists from the Institute for Aerobics Research and the Cooper Clinic in Dallas divided a population of 13,344 men and women into five categories of fitness, ranging from sedentary people to well-conditioned athletes. Predictably, those who exercised the least died the soonest. However, the scientists were surprised to find that the greatest health benefit was derived by those who simply got out and walked for half an hour a day, three or four times a week, which cut their chances of having a heart attack or developing cancer by more than half.

To borrow a familiar phrase, exercise "is the right thing to do." And you don't have to do a lot of it, as long as you do it on a regular basis, week in and week out.

## YOUR PERSONAL EXERCISE PRESCRIPTION

The most common aerobic exercises include walking, running, swimming, jumping rope, cross-country skiing, stair climbing and aerobic dance. Many competitive sports, such as basketball, soccer, tennis and racquetball, are also aerobic if pursued for sustained amounts of time.

To benefit from an aerobic program, you should exercise for at least 15 to 20 minutes a day, three or four days a week. You have to work hard enough to get your heart rate up between 60 and 85 percent of its maximum, according to the American College of Sports Medicine.

So how do you figure this? To estimate your maximal heart rate, subtract your age from 220. If you are 40 years old, for example, your maximal heart rate would be around 180. To get the greatest aerobic benefit from an exercise session, then, you should get your heart rate up between 108 and 153 beats per minute, and keep it there for 15 to 20 minutes. However, there is evidence that many exercise benefits can occur at heart rates slightly below this target range as well.

To find your heart rate, use your middle and index fingers to measure your pulse at your wrist. Count the number of beats for 15 seconds, and multiply by four.

It's very important that you warm up before you begin any workout. Walk at a leisurely pace or pedal slowly to prepare your muscles, heart and respiratory system for your workout. After a five- or ten-minute warm-up, do some light stretching. Once you've finished your workout, cool down with a few minutes of walking or gentle stretching to allow your heart to resume its normal cadence.

## DISCOVER THE SIMPLEST OF PLEASURES

Walking is one of the best exercises anyone can do, and it's probably the best choice if you're out of shape to start with.

For David Balboa, sports psychotherapist and co-director of New York's Walking Center, there's walking, and then there's the *art* of walking. "Walking should feel like a gentle massage," he says. "Walk as smoothly as possible, trying to sustain a gliding, effortless motion." Most of us walk from the hips down, says Balboa, which increases the tension in our hips and pelvis and leads to fatigue and low-back pain. Here's how to improve your walking style and increase your enjoyment of this pleasant activity.

**Roll from heel to toe.** Concentrate on placing your heel on the ground, and allow your foot to roll from heel to toe. "While your foot rolls, feel the ground with your foot," explains Balboa. "By concentrating on this action, you will naturally straighten your leg when you take a step and walk, which will correct your posture from the ground up."

**Move your torso.** Don't just step from below your waist; imagine that your torso, hip and leg are united in a fluid motion in which all three move forward together. "Most people walk as if their pelvis is a rigid block," says Balboa. "It's the old John Wayne–style of walking—he never moved his hips. But that creates a lot of tension in the pelvis. Allow your pelvis to roll naturally as you walk. Imagine that your leg motion begins a few inches above your belly button; then your side, hip and leg will move smoothly together. This position will automatically improve your posture and allow your hips to move naturally as you walk."

**Relax your shoulders.** Shoulders should be relaxed and dropped. "Don't walk as if you're carrying a bag of groceries," Balboa says. "Let your arms hang and swing naturally."

**Choose a scenic route.** "Pick an area you'll enjoy walking in, a place that will take your mind off the exercise," says Robert E. Goldman, D.O., Ph.D., director of the National Academy of Sports Medicine in Chicago. Also, vary the locations. Hike in different parks, neighborhoods or woods.

**Walk with others.** Once you have improved your conditioning, join a walking club, says Dr. Cisar. "Walking with friends, especially on long hikes, can be a lot of fun."

## GET IN THE SWIM

Swimming remains one of the most popular sports and an excellent fitness activity. A half-hour of swimming will give you a whole-body aerobic workout and burn anywhere from 150 to 300 calories, depending on how hard you push yourself. Here are some tips to improve your workout.

**Stretch out first.** Warming up before swimming increases blood flow and flexibility. Perform shoulder rolls, head turns, trunk turns and hamstring stretches, either in or out of the water.

**Learn a different stroke.** Doing the crawl lap after lap can eventually bore even a devout swimmer. Find an instructor or pick up a book on swimming, and try the backstroke, breaststroke, sidestroke or butterfly.

**Streamline your swimming.** If you're in decent shape but feel winded after a lap or two, your style may be the problem, says Jane Katz, Ed.D., former Olympic swimmer, professor of physical education at the City University of New York and author of *The W.E.T. Workout* and *Swim 30 Laps in 30 Days*. Many people swing or jerk their heads excessively while swimming, thrash their arms wildly or just don't have the hang of breathing correctly.

**Try out accessories.** To make your workout more effective and fun, use pull buoys, hand paddles or kick boards. Pull buoys are pieces of Styrofoam that fit between your legs and hold them up in the water so you can concentrate on your arms. Kick boards help you improve your kick, while hand paddles increase your upper-body effort and enhance your swimming technique. Some paddles, for example, are designed to improve hand entry into the water and to fully extend your push.

## WORK OUT WET—WITHOUT THE SWEAT

You'd love to work out in the water, but you can't swim, or you hate the grind of lap swimming? "You don't have to be a good swimmer to enjoy a wet workout," says Dr. Katz. "You can walk or 'run' back and forth in the shallow end of a swimming pool or do a variety of water calisthenics, and get a great aerobic workout."

Water reduces the gravitational force on the body. When you're in chin-deep water, for example, you weigh one-tenth what you normally do. At chest deep, you're about one-third of your weight; at waist deep, about half. This takes the strain off joints and bones, making water aerobics great for people with arthritis, back problems or bone, joint and muscular disorders. Water workouts are also great for overweight people and for pregnant women.

Water provides 12 times the resistance that air provides, with variable resistance: The harder you push against the water, the more resistance it offers. Dr. Katz recommends calisthenics in waist- and chest-deep water. Do each exercise for about 5 minutes; the workout should take from 20 to 30 minutes for full aerobic benefit. Some sample exercises:

**Circle your arms.** In shoulder-deep water, extend your arms outward and rotate them in small circles. Do these clockwise, then counter-clockwise. Gradually make the circles larger.

**Lift those legs.** Stand with your back to the corner of the pool, your arms on the edge for support. Lift up your legs until they're parallel to the bottom of the pool. (You are now in a sitting position, with your legs extended.) Put your legs together and slowly turn them to the extreme left and right.

**Jump to it.** In waist- or chest-deep water, do jumping jacks. From a standing position with your arms at your sides, simultaneously jump outward with your legs and clap your hands over your head. Wear a lifejacket to keep you upright and prevent you from going under if you slip.

**Walk in water.** In the shallow end of the pool, walk or run. Or wear a flotation vest and run in the deep end.

### TENNIS FOR FUN AND FITNESS

Tennis, anyone? Not only is this a fun game, it's a valuable aerobic activity. Researchers discovered that tennis players tend to be lean and in good aerobic shape. Of course, if you just lazily bat the ball around, stroll to pick up the ones you miss and pause to chat, you won't get much of a workout. But an active game works plenty of muscles as well as the heart and lungs. To make tennis even more aerobically rewarding, you can try the following strategies.

**Hustle for the ball.** Run down every ball, even those you don't think you can get. (Look what it's done for Jimmy Connors.) Hurry after the ones you miss; when you pick up a ball, bend your knees and stretch for it.

**Move behind it.** Make a point of getting behind an oncoming ball, rather than hitting it when it's already at your side. This will improve your technique, power and workout.

**Bend those knees.** Bend your knees for every shot, and then raise your body as your racket approaches the ball. This puts topspin on the ball and exercises your legs. Also, follow through on every shot to give your game more power and your body a better workout. Follow-through will also protect you against tennis elbow, or inflammation of the tendons of the forearm.

**Use your imagination.** Play "shadow tennis," developed by former Davis Cup captain Dennis Ralston. Pick out an imaginary opponent and beat the pants off him or her. Don't let up. Stretch for serves, overheads and slams; follow through on backhands and forehands; bend your knees; and move around the court as quickly as you can. Start with one-minute workouts and work your way to five minutes. This is also a great way to warm up before a match.

## REMEMBER OTHER RACKET SPORTS

Tennis isn't the only racket sport—racquetball, squash and badminton are good aerobic options, too. Racquetball and squash are especially intense because you play against walls, which makes the game fast and keeps the ball in play longer. A player can burn between 600 and 850 calories an hour.

For playing these three sports on the competitive level, doctors recommend wearing protective, shatterproof goggles with polycarbonate plastic lenses. The lenses in regular eyeglasses won't withstand the impact of a ball moving at speeds that can exceed 140 miles an hour.

**Pick up racquetball.** The beauty of the game is that you can pick up the basics so quickly that you can play right away.

And because you're hitting the ball almost constantly, you're getting a great workout.

**Give squash a whirl.** Squash is played with a smaller, less bouncy ball and a longer racket with a smaller head than used for racquetball. It's tougher to learn and demands good physical condition. If you're in shape and want a mental challenge, this may be the sport for you.

**Try out badminton.** Yes, the lawn variety will give you a gentle workout, but if you want something more taxing, you can try indoor badminton. It burns about 350 calories an hour, and 20 minutes of playing incorporates lots of running, jumping and stretching.

*Editor's note:* The quick lateral movements required in tennis and other racket sports can result in injuries, including sprains and tears, to unstable joints and unconditioned muscles. If you're out of shape or have weak knees or ankles, you should strengthen your muscles and ligaments with resistance training before trying these sports. (See chapter 32.)

## BRING YOUR PROGRAM INDOORS

A stationary cycle, treadmill, cross-country ski machine or step-climbing machine can provide an outstanding aerobic workout, either in your own home or at a health club. A 170-pound man who rides an exercise bike for 20 minutes at 20 miles an hour will burn 200 calories, for example. He'll get a great aerobic workout that will exercise his entire lower body. A similar session on a stair climber or treadmill will burn roughly the same number of calories as cycling, while adding variety to your workout.

Dr. Goldman points out that using step-climbing and treadmill equipment prevents what he calls the ballistic injuries that result from the shock of impact when your foot hits the ground while walking or running. Keep these tips in mind if you're putting together a home exercise program.

**Shop carefully.** Exercise machines vary in quality, so shop around before buying. Ask friends or personnel at health clubs for recommendations. It's also a good idea to try out the machine before you take it home.

**Choose a strategic position.** "I tell people to put the stationary cycle or treadmill in front of the television," says Dr. Goldman. "That way, you're entertained while you work out, and the exercise equipment is in a place where you can't miss it."

**Put on some tunes.** A study published in the *Journal of Sports & Exercise Psychology* shows that people who exercise to music are like the Energizer rabbit—they keep going and going, while those who exercise without listening to music stop sooner. Music makes the workout more fun, and because you are distracted, you can keep going a bit longer.

## TAKE OFF ON SKIS

When it comes to aerobic activities, cross-country skiing ranks high. It gives a nearly total-body workout and burns lots of calories to boot. This sport works the shoulders, arms, chest, abdomen, buttocks and legs. Studies have shown that an hour of cross-country skiing will burn between 600 and 900 calories. Champion cross-country skiers have burned as many as 1,000 calories an hour and reached the highest levels of $VO_2$ max ever recorded. And rather than causing injuries, cross-country skiing has been shown to strengthen joints and bones.

**Take a lesson.** While you can rent skis and go out on your own, unless you are remarkably physically adept, you'll probably end up just shuffling along on the skis, not getting a great workout and not having much fun, either. After just one or two lessons, however, you can master the kick-and-glide routine.

**Dress appropriately.** You don't need the bulky, heavily insulated clothing required for downhill skiing. Instead, dress in layers: long underwear, outer clothing and wind pants and a jacket on top. Add wool socks, gloves, a hat and a neck covering, and you're set.

**Sample a machine.** Yes, a quality cross-country machine—not a $75 special—will provide a workout nearly identical to the outdoor variety. Try out a ski machine before you commit yourself, however, because some people find them tough to master. "The quality of the aerobic workout depends on whether you feel comfortable on the machine so that you can get your heart rate up to the target zone and stay with it long enough to condition yourself," says Dr. Cisar.

## ANTI-AGING CHECKUP
# RATING YOUR EFFORT

It's generally a good idea to get your physician's okay before starting an exercise program, particularly if you're over 35. And anyone with a history of heart disease or with a major risk factor, such as smoking or elevated blood pressure or cholesterol, *must* check with a physician.

Once you begin your program, you'll want to monitor the intensity of your exertion. The simplest way to make sure you're not overdoing it is the "speak" test: Can you speak while you're exercising? If you can't talk as you work out, your intensity is too high.

Or you can keep tabs on your heart rate. Is it within 60 to 90 percent of your maximum? (Your maximum is approximately 220 minus your age.) For those just starting a program, 60 percent is adequate to condition your heart, respiratory and musculoskeletal system.

Another way to rate your effort is the Borg Rate of Perceived Exertion Scale. Studies have shown that your perception of how strenuously you are working out closely correlates with your heart rate and other metabolic processes that occur during exercise. When you say you've reached a 5 on a scale of 1 to 10, studies indicate that you are accurately perceiving that your heart rate and muscle exertion have reached half their max.

### BORG'S SCALE

| | | | |
|---|---|---|---|
| 0 | Nothing at all | 5 | Strong (heavy) |
| 0.5 | Very, very weak | 6 | |
| | (just noticeable) | 7 | Very strong |
| 1 | Very weak | 8 | |
| 2 | Weak (light) | 9 | |
| 3 | Moderate | 10 | Very, very strong |
| 4 | Somewhat strong | | (almost max) |

Safety is always the first concern in all types of exercise, however. Listen to your body, learn your limits, and be very careful whenever you attempt to move beyond what you know you can do.

# 2

# ANGINA

## How to Keep the Pain Away

**If** anything can be characterized as the grip of death, then certainly angina pectoris—which literally means "strangling" in the chest—qualifies. Angina is the heart muscle crying out for enough oxygen from the blood to keep pumping.

It's caused by cholesterol plaques clogging the arteries that lead to the heart, or by spasms of arteries at the site of these plaques. When an oxygen-starved heart is forced to beat faster during exercise, under stress or in extreme heat or cold, the stage is set for an angina attack. That's because the heart muscle, when forced to exert itself, needs added oxygen to meet the challenge. But when the coronary arteries are partially blocked, the blood can't get through to deliver the oxygen the heart needs. The result is a constricting pain, often severe, that can spread from the chest to the throat, upper jaw, back and left arm and usually lasts five to ten minutes.

Other common angina triggers include cigarette smoking, which deprives cells of oxygen; being overweight; eating a big meal; strong emotional reactions; and the dream stage of sleep.

No question about it, angina pain is heavy-duty pain—and it is a sign that you may be at risk of heart attack. No wonder an episode of angina is quick to get a physician's undivided attention. Nevertheless, it's reassuring to know that angina can be prevented. Furthermore, many of those who already suffer from the disease can make a full recovery.

### Exercise May Leave Pain Behind

True, strenuous exercise can bring on an angina attack, but steady, moderate exercise below angina-inducing levels can be a remedy for the illness. A study published in the *American Journal of Cardiology* reported lower incidence of angina pain and improved circulation to the heart resulting from a daily regimen of simple calisthenics.

Forty men with angina were divided into two groups, one of which did not exercise. The other followed the Canadian Air Force program of 11 minutes a day of calisthenics that required no weights or equipment. Within eight weeks, the exercisers experienced a significant reduction of angina pain. In fact, 6 of those 20 men saw all their symptoms disappear during those eight weeks. By the end of the study, the exercise group's blood flow to the heart had improved more than 30 percent, which translated into fewer angina attacks.

Calisthenics aren't the only option, however. Walking is the best exercise for angina patients, says Paul D. Thompson, M.D., director of the Cardiovascular Disease Prevention Center at the University of Pittsburgh Heart Institute. "I tell people to walk as far as they can until they encounter pain. That's their threshold distance," he says. "Then take a nitroglycerin pill (which increases the blood flow through the heart muscle and the whole body) and rest. After the pain has passed, walk back home. Do that three to five times a week, and you will see the threshold distances get longer and longer before you experience any pain." You should, of course, check with your doctor before beginning any exercise program, and it's crucial that you do so if you have pain at rest, or pain that lasts more than five minutes after taking nitroglycerin.

### Four More Angina-Fighting Strategies

Besides exercise, there are other steps you can take to reduce the risk of suffering angina. Here are a few.

**Cut dietary fat.** Atherosclerosis, or clogged arteries, is caused by high blood cholesterol levels. Most people can lower these by restricting the amount of fat and cholesterol in the diet. That will improve your circulation and slow the underlying cause of angina, says Dr. Thompson. (See chapters 8 and 19.)

---

**ANTI-AGING CHECKUP**
## ANGINA SIGNALS YOU CAN'T MISS

Some people dismiss angina as indigestion or other harmless chest pains; others worry that every chest pain is dangerous. If you suspect you're having an attack, pay attention to the following symptoms, which may signal angina.

_____ Feelings of heaviness
_____ A burning sensation in your chest
_____ A sense of pressure in your chest
_____ An instinctive urge to press a closed fist or open hand against your chest while experiencing pain
_____ Pain lasting five to ten minutes, just below your breast-bone, radiating out through the shoulders, neck, jaw and arm, and most often the left arm
_____ Weakness and tightness in your chest, plus shortness of breath
_____ A pain in your chest that awakens you from sleep
_____ A sudden sense of exhaustion during exercise that forces you to stop at once

### INTERPRETING YOUR ANSWERS

If you experience _any_ of these symptoms, contact a physician as soon as possible for a professional evaluation of your condition.

---

**Eat more whole grains and produce.** Replace the fatty foods in your diet with whole grains, fresh vegetables and fruit. Many of these foods are rich in vitamins C and E and beta-carotene, which researchers say may reduce the incidence and severity of angina.

A study published in the British medical journal _Lancet_ showed that higher blood levels of vitamins C and E and beta-carotene were associated with significantly fewer angina attacks. Conversely, the same study disclosed that low blood levels of vitamin E were associated with more than twice the risk of angina.

**Lighten your heart's burden.** Obesity can be deadly for anyone, but particularly for people who suffer from angina. According to Michael Weber, M.D., professor of medicine at the University of California, Irvine, College of Medicine, the excess pounds increase the burden on the heart by elevating blood pressure, which encourages fat-deposit buildup in the arteries. The increased pressure on the protective inner lining of the wall creates fissures and cracks, where LDL cholesterol gains a foothold and forms cholesterol plaques that add up to atherosclerosis. Losing weight should be a gradual program that combines exercise with healthier eating habits, including fewer fats and more whole grains, fruits and vegetables. (See chapter 27 for detailed tips.)

**Ask your doctor about aspirin.** Plain old aspirin prevents blood platelets from forming the clots that can cut off blood flow to the heart. "For those who have already had vascular disease, either heart attack, angina or stroke, there is conclusive evidence that low-dose aspirin decreases the risk of subsequent stroke, heart attack or death," says Charles Henneken, M.D., acting chairman of preventive medicine at Harvard Medical School.

But because some evidence suggests that those who take aspirin to prevent a first heart attack may slightly increase their risk of suffering a stroke, doctors advise heart patients to take aspirin only with the approval of a physician.

# 3

# ARTHRITIS

## Simple Ways to Limber Up

You may have watched a parent or grandparent grow stiff from arthritis and accepted the condition as an inevitable, painful part of aging. For centuries, temporary pain relief was the best anyone could hope for.

But times have changed. There are plenty of things you can do to fight and maybe even help prevent arthritis. Research offers a host of promising new therapies that not only control most of the symptoms but also hold out the hope that one day this disease can be defeated completely.

The key to dealing with arthritis is not letting it control your life but creating a program to maximize your improvement and help you deal with the problem. That program, say the experts, includes exercise, external treatments (massage, compresses, wraps and such), proper diet, rest and medication when needed. A variety of medications are available, ranging from simple aspirin to nonsteroidal anti-inflammatory drugs (NSAIDs).

One thing is certain: Arthritis needn't be a crippling disease. With the right program and a little perseverance, you can take charge of arthritis. "The first thing you have to do is understand the type of arthritis you have and then what treatments work best for you," says Harris H. McIlwain, M.D., a rheumatologist and joint expert practicing in Tampa and one of the authors of *Winning with Arthritis*.

*Editor's note:* Treatment—including medication and physical therapy—can differ for everyone, so it's important to work with your doctor to find the right program for you. It's also best to see a doctor as soon as you suspect you have arthritis so you can begin treatment early.

## BONE UP ON WHAT ARTHRITIS REALLY IS

Arthritis, which means inflammation of the joints, affects about 34 million Americans of all ages. It can attack any joint and cause pain, swelling, stiffness, a sensation of heat at the affected parts and, less commonly, deformity. In addition, some forms of arthritis cause a wide range of seemingly unrelated symptoms, including fatigue, fever, skin rash, mouth sores, hair loss, diarrhea and heart, liver and kidney disorders.

Arthritis is not one disease but more than a hundred. The most common forms are osteoarthritis, which causes the cartilage in the joints to degenerate; rheumatoid arthritis, also know as inflammatory arthritis because it is associated with severe swelling of joints and other tissues; and gout, which is caused by uric acid collecting in the joints.

Though scientists still have not pinpointed the specific causes of arthritis, they do know that rheumatoid arthritis, the most severe form, is an autoimmune disease: It causes the body's own immune system to attack the tissues of the joints. Osteoarthritis, the most common form, usually afflicts the weight-bearing joints—the knees, hips and spine. Athletes who injure a joint often develop osteoarthritis in the affected area, and the illness is more common in overweight people. All of this suggests that osteoarthritis is associated with excessive wear and tear of bones and connective tissues.

## GET THE JUMP ON ACHING JOINTS

Don't wait for aching joints to take over your life before you begin to fight back. If you hurt at all, start today to ease your discomfort, using a few simple nondrug remedies.

**Apply moist heat.** Hot, moist towels, a shower, a bath or a whirlpool are ideal ways to loosen stiff and painful joints. Treat with heat in the mornings, when stiffness is most common, and evenings, when joints sometimes tighten as a result of the day's demands. Though dry heating pads may be more convenient, moist heat is more effective because it stimulates circulation and flexibility and makes exercise easier. That's why many people apply hot compresses in combination with an exercise routine. Your physician or medical-supply store can provide you with ready-made hot packs called hydrocollator packs.

**Use cold compresses.** To reduce swelling, especially when it occurs at the end of the day, apply a cold pack or ice. Cold reduces swelling, while heat relaxes muscles and stimulates circulation. Consequently, many people combine the two: They apply moist heat for about 15 minutes, followed by a cold compress for another 15 minutes. Experiment to see what works best for you.

**Keep those joints moving.** People with arthritis are understandably reluctant to flex achy joints. But when joints don't get much use, the muscles weaken and shrink. When muscle mass is lost, greater pressure is placed on the bones and cartilage, which causes even more pain and degeneration. Thus, one of the most important things people with arthritis can do is to keep their muscles strong and conditioned.

"If I could choose only one treatment for arthritis, it would be exercise, even over medication," says Dr. McIlwain. "Exercise is one of the most underused treatments available today and one of the most important. By maintaining an exercise program, you make the muscles in the joints flexible, limber and strong, which supports the joints and reduces the pain." Exercise can be used for all the leading forms of arthritis, including osteoarthritis, rheumatoid and gout.

## STAY LOOSE

Dr. McIlwain and his coauthors offer a wide variety of exercises in *Winning with Arthritis*. These and other exercises not only strengthen muscles and increase muscle mass, they help joints become looser and more flexible, thus allowing greater range of motion without pain. "The big thing is that you do these exercises properly and consistently," says Dr. McIlwain. "Many people who exercise regularly will be able to avoid medication altogether." These warm-ups will loosen you up for more specialized movements.

**Breathe deeply.** Lie on your back, with your hands placed comfortably behind your head and your knees bent. Breathe deeply, raising your chest while filling your lungs completely. Hold for about 2 seconds, and then exhale by drawing in your abdomen. Start slowly. Do 5 repetitions, gradually increasing to 10 and then 20.

**Flex your back.** Lie on your back, knees bent, your feet flat on the floor and your hands stretched out toward the ceiling. Now move your arms and turn your head to the right, while your knees move to the left. Reverse the above and then repeat. Do 5 repetitions and gradually work your way up to 10.

**Bicycle on your back.** Lie on your back. Lift your legs, knees bent, into the air and pedal in slow, rhythmic movements, as though bicycling. Count to 6 and then relax. That's one complete exercise. Do 5 repetitions and gradually increase to 10.

### RESISTANCE EXERCISES FOR THE SHOULDERS

It's good to challenge your shoulder muscles regularly through simple exercises so joints remain supple and pain-free in everyday activities. Add these to your daily routine.

*Editor's note:* If weight-bearing exercise is painful for you, you should first strengthen your muscles and ligaments through resistance training. (See chapter 32.) Your doctor can also recommend exercises.

**Work those wrists.** Loop a rubber band designed for exercise over both wrists, then pull your arms (held stiff) as far apart as you can. Hold the tension for 5 seconds and then relax.

**Now pull up and down.** With the rubber band in the same position, place one arm above the other and then move the upper arm up and the lower arm down until the rubber band is taut. Hold the tension for 5 seconds. Release and repeat with your hands in the opposite positions.

**Stretch behind you.** Hold the rubber band with one hand behind your head and the other behind your back. Stretch the rubber band as far as you can and hold it for 5 seconds. Release and reverse hands to repeat the exercise.

# TRACKING CLUES TO A POSSIBLE CURE

Imagine controlling your arthritis by . . . not medication but what you eat. Scientists have suspected for some time that diet has a connection to arthritis, and research has indicated that very simple diets and even fasting can curb symptoms. In one study reported in the British medical journal *Lancet,* for example, scientists in Norway compared two groups of people suffering from rheumatoid arthritis. One group of 27 people followed an experimental vegetarian diet, while a control group of 26 followed a standard diet.

The vegetarian diet comprised three stages. The first lasted seven to ten days and included vegetable broths, vegetable juices, herbal teas and garlic. The second stage, which lasted 3½ months, consisted entirely of vegetable foods, with no red meat, eggs, dairy foods, citrus fruits, refined sugars, spices, salt or grains containing gluten. After 4 months, dairy foods were introduced one at a time, with a new product allowed every other day. That final diet was followed for one year. Both groups kept diaries of their eating habits and noted any symptoms.

The results of the study were startling. After one month, the experimental group experienced significant decreases in the number of swollen and tender joints, how long morning stiffness lasted and a number of other parameters that indicate arthritis flare-ups. The experimental group also felt stronger and healthier overall. Remarkably, these gains were maintained over the 13-month duration of the study.

The control group felt less pain during the first four weeks, but their blood values did not improve. By the end of the study, all the symptoms—including pain—had worsened for the control group.

The researchers concluded, "We have shown that in some patients a substantial reduction in disease activity can be obtained by fasting followed by an individually adjusted vegetarian diet." Thus far, however, the effect of diet on arthritis is still very speculative.

## RESISTANCE EXERCISES FOR ELBOWS AND HIPS

When you bend over to pick up the morning paper, you're quickly reminded of any stiff and creaky joints you might have in your arms and torso. The following moves can help loosen up those areas.

**Stretch the elbows.** With a rubber band designed for exercise looped around your wrists, hold out your left arm directly in front of you while pulling your right arm toward your chest. Hold for 5 seconds, then repeat, with your right arm out in front of you while you draw the left toward your chest.

**Take to the water.** Swimming and wet workouts are also good exercises for arthritis because water reduces the body weight—thus placing less stress on joints—while providing excellent resistance for your muscles to work against.

## DANCE YOUR WAY TO PAIN RELIEF AND FLEXIBILITY

Dancing, an activity reluctantly abandoned by many people with arthritis, is catching on as an exercise therapy to increase ease of movement. Milton Feher, who opened the Milton Feher School of Dance and Relaxation in New York in 1945, teaches people with arthritis to dance away stiffness and pain.

"Every motion you do, you can turn into a dance," says Feher. "It teaches you how the different parts of the body relate to each other. Everyone who wants to use his or her body better has to learn that."

While you may not find a program designed specifically for people with arthritis, you can join any dance class or social club and participate as much as you can. Dancing a waltz, square dance, swing beat or salsa rhythm can be a fun way to loosen joints, strengthen muscles and let go of pain.

Before you put on your dancing shoes—or begin any kind of exercise program—check with your doctor. Many people with arthritis also suffer from cardiovascular disease, which, if stressed by excessive exercise, can bring on a heart attack or stroke. The best approach is to start slowly and gradually build up your fitness and endurance.

## ANTI-AGING CHECKUP
# WHY ARE YOUR JOINTS THUMPING?

Painful knees, elbows or shoulders can make you feel as old as Methuselah long before you qualify for seniors' rates at the movies. Arthritis pain might strike at any age, and the discomfort can be just as intense at 35 as at 60.

But every bout you have with aching joints doesn't mean arthritis. A hard bump, an overenthusiastic game of tennis or a weekend spent chasing after a toddler when you're out of shape can leave you with knees or shoulders that hurt like blazes! But these pains may have nothing to do with arthritis.

So when should you suspect arthritis? The Arthritis Foundation recommends seeing a physician if you experience pain, swelling, stiffness or problems in using one or more joints for two weeks or longer. And if you do see a doctor, here's what you can expect to be asked as the doctor probes for further clues. To help your doctor make a diagnosis, be prepared with your answers.

_____ Which joints hurt, and how long have they bothered you?

_____ Do the painful joints swell or feel hot inside?

_____ Is there a time—early morning, after work, bedtime— when the pain is particularly bad?

_____ What, if anything, makes your joints feel better or worse?

_____ Are there any other symptoms—fever, weight loss, rashes, fatigue, dry eyes or mouth, pain in other joints, nausea or diarrhea?

_____ Does anyone in your family have arthritis?

## INTERPRETING YOUR ANSWERS

If you're lucky, your discomfort may simply be due to a bruise or too much unaccustomed activity. If, on the other hand, you do have arthritis of some sort, you can still live with minimum pain and maximum flexibility by exercising regularly, improving your diet and getting proper medical care. Start now.

## DISCOVER THE DIFFERENCE DIET CAN MAKE

Ninety percent of those who suffer from arthritis try some form of alternative therapy, and the most common one is diet.

Scientists agree that changes in diet may affect arthritis. After an extensive review of scientific evidence, L. Gail Darlington, M.D., concluded in an article in Rheumatic Disease Clinics of North America that dietary therapy may be useful for at least some people with rheumatoid arthritis. Two of the most popular therapies include the use of fish oil or vitamins.

Fish oil—omega-3 polyunsaturated fatty acids containing eicosapentaenoic acid (EPA)—apparently has an anti-inflammatory effect on rheumatoid arthritis patients. In one six-month study, Joel Kremer, M.D., a professor of medicine at Albany Medical College in New York, compared the effects of fish oils and olive oil on 49 people with rheumatoid arthritis. Dr. Kremer found that the standard symptoms of inflammation—pain, stiffness and fatigue, were significantly lower in those taking fish-oil capsules than in those taking olive oil. Moreover, he discovered that increasing the doses of fish oil decreased symptoms even more.

Another study, reported in the British medical journal *Lancet,* showed that people with osteoarthritis also experienced relief of pain and greater flexibility after increasing their intake of fish oil for six months.

Fish oil isn't for everyone, however. People with diabetes or who have a tendency to bleed or hemorrhage should use fish oil only with their physician's recommendation. *Eating* more oily fish—such as salmon, tuna, halibut and sardines—is safer than taking capsules.

And doses of vitamins may help. Vitamins A, C and E may reduce the pain, swelling and other symptoms of arthritis, according to Arthur I. Grayzel, M.D., medical director at the Arthritis Foundation in Atlanta. These vitamins are antioxidants, which can neutralize harmful loose oxygen molecules in your body called free radicals.

"There is some evidence that free radicals may contribute to the symptoms of arthritis and that the antioxidants may reduce free radical formation," says Dr. Grayzel. Beta-carotene, the vegetable source of vitamin A, is abundant in leafy greens (collard greens, broccoli and kale), root vegetables (carrots and rutabagas), brussels sprouts and squash. Vitamin E appears in whole grains and seafoods, while C is abundant in citrus fruits, cabbage, leafy greens, broccoli and peppers, among many other foods.

"A lot is unknown about diet yet. Much more research has to be done," comments Dr. McIlwain. "Arthritis research is still very young." You should check with your doctor before making any major changes in your diet.

# 4

# BACK AND
# NECK PAIN

### Staying in the Game

It can happen suddenly. You're playing a weekend game of softball with your kids or maybe just bending down to pick up the morning newspaper. Zap! Pain rips through your lower back and down your legs as if someone had plunged a knife into your kidney.

Or it can happen gradually, with pain slowly creeping into the ligaments, muscles and vertebrae until it grips your lower back.

Regardless of how back or neck pain strikes, it can be excruciating and disabling, lasting days, weeks or even months. And it doesn't just happen to any unlucky few. By some estimates, 80 percent of us suffer from back pain at one time or another. Yet experts tell us that most back pain is completely preventable, and even chronic and debilitating pain can be overcome.

"By doing some regular exercises that improve strength and flexibility, most back pain can be avoided," says Willibald Nagler, M.D., chief physiatrist at New York Hospital, Cornell Medical College. "Prevention is the key to keeping yourself from suffering from back pain."

To Find Solutions, Examine the Causes

Back pain arises from a variety of causes. Among the most common:

- jobs that involve repetitive motion, such as laying bricks or working on an assembly line
- trauma from car accidents or sports-related injuries
- degeneration of muscles, ligaments and tissues of the back and abdomen, resulting in the inability to provide support
- arthritis
- osteoporosis
- stress, which can cause muscles in the back to go into spasm and pull on vertebrae

Other factors could also be involved, such as sitting at a desk or driving a car for hours without stopping, poor posture and even drinking excess alcohol or smoking cigarettes, which are risk factors for osteoporosis. Scientists theorize that compounds in cigarette smoke may also interfere with the ability of vertebral disks to absorb nutrients, thus leading to degeneration.

For most people who suffer from back pain, however, all of these factors boil down to a single cause: taut muscles.

"Excess muscle tension means that particular muscles are working too hard, for too long," explains physical therapist Mike Hage in *The Back Pain Book: A Self-Help Guide for Daily Relief of Neck and Back Pain.* "Excess muscle tension pulls and crams joints together. This increased compression can trigger off pain circuits along the spine, and this can cause increased pain not only in the neck and low back but in the arms and legs as well."

That's also how emotional stress causes back pain. "When you feel angry, anxious, tired, ill or depressed, your brain automatically increases your sensitivity to pain," writes Hage. "Feelings of fear, anger or anxiety tend to increase muscle tension around the face and head and along the spine. This crams joints together and overworks your muscles, aggravating your pain."

As vertebrae compress, the disks in between can bulge or slip, a condition called a herniated disk. Once a disk goes out of alignment, it can press against the sciatic nerve that runs along the spinal column and down the leg. The sciatic nerve is that all-too-familiar pain circuit that lights up whenever back pain flares.

Eighty-five million Americans suffer from back pain, according to Leonard Faye, D.C., a chiropractor and author of *Good-Bye Back Pain!* Each year, more than 240,000 victims of back pain undergo surgery, but according to Dr. Faye, only 2 to 3 percent of those who suffer chronic back pain really need surgery.

The secret to preventing and overcoming back pain, say the experts, lies in dealing with tension and strengthening muscles that support the back.

### STRETCH AWAY THE PAIN

Because most back pain is caused by either weak back and abdominal muscles or compression on nerves and disks (or both), the best treatment involves strengthening the back and abdomen and relieving tension through a variety of stretching exercises.

The following exercises, outlined in Dr. Faye's book, have been effective for many people with chronic back pain. These movements will stretch ligaments and muscles, making them stronger, more flexible and better coordinated. You should see improvement in your range of motion and a diminishing of pain within a month, according to Dr. Faye.

You can easily hurt cold muscles, so it's best to warm them up a bit before you start to stretch. One good way is to take a ten-minute walk before you begin. Remember to start stretching gently and slowly, and stop any exercise that causes sharp pain or pain that lingers. If you feel a dull ache or pain, however, try to relax into it and allow it to pass.

Attempt to hold each of the following stretches for about 25 to 30 seconds (unless otherwise indicated), and do the exercises daily for about 20 minutes. Be sure to breathe regularly and easily, exhaling for the last 5 seconds of each exercise.

**Lean into it.** Sit on a chair and lean forward. At the point where you begin to feel pain, breathe out and try to relax into the pain slightly. This will stretch the spine and back muscles and ligaments.

**Pull your knee.** Sit upright in a straight-backed chair. Lift your right knee up and take hold of it with both hands, pulling it toward your chest until it's up as high as possible. Repeat with the left leg.

**Stretch your pelvis.** Take the same position as in the previous exercise. Lift your right leg toward your chest by grasping your knee, and move the knee gently toward your left shoulder. This stretches the pelvis and lumbar muscles even farther than the previous exercise. Repeat the stretch, this time moving your left knee toward your right shoulder.

**Push your thigh.** Sit in a chair and place your right foot on your left thigh, near the knee. Gently push your inner right knee and thigh down toward the floor, stretching your groin and lower back muscles. Repeat, using the left leg.

**Pull your ankle.** Stand behind a straight-backed chair and hold on to it for support. Take hold of your right ankle with your right hand and pull your leg back until your heel touches your right buttock. Repeat, using the left ankle. If you are able, add more stretch by moving your knee backward.

**Stretch lying down.** Lie on your back on the floor or a firm mat. With both hands, take hold of your right knee and pull it toward your chest. Repeat with the other leg.

**Do both at once.** Lying down, take hold of your knees. Bring both legs up to your chest.

**Rotate those knees.** Lie on your back, bending your knees while keeping your feet on the floor. Rotate your knees to the right, bringing them toward the floor, while turning your head to the left as far as you can. Then reverse the motion: Rotate your knees to the left and your head to the right.

**Lift your buns.** Lie on your back, bending your knees while keeping your feet on the floor. Gently lift your buttocks as high as you can and hold for a count of 8. Repeat the exercise as many times as you can without overdoing it; gradually work your way to 10 repetitions without pain.

**Touch your forehead.** Get down on your hands and knees. Lift your right knee off the floor and bring it to your forehead. (Do not force it if you cannot touch your forehead.) Now push your right leg backward until you can stretch the leg straight out, parallel to the floor. Bring your knee back to the floor, and repeat the exercise with the left leg.

As a variation on this exercise, raise your right arm and point it straight out in front of you while your left leg is raised and pointing straight back. Reverse the position: left arm out, right leg up and straight back.

### To Save Your Back, Work the Abs

Your belly might be the biggest problem your lower back has to contend with. "When the stomach (abdominal) muscles are weak and the stomach is expanded," says Dr. Nagler, "it forces the spine and lower-back muscles to carry an extra load. This makes the lower back more vulnerable to injury."

Research has shown that the lower backs of people with chronic back problems were as strong as those with healthy backs. The difference was that those with weak abdominal muscles had more back problems than those with stronger abdominal muscles. In a study in the *Journal of New Developments in Clinical Medicine,* 82 percent of the 233 participants either had no back pain whatsoever or much less pain after they started to exercise regularly.

To improve abdominal strength, do crunch sit-ups, says Wayne Westcott, Ph.D., YMCA national strength-training consultant in Arlington, Massachusetts. You want to avoid a full sit-up, where you sit all the way up, which exercises the hips and legs more than the abdomen and could strain your back.

Start on your back with your knees bent, feet flat on the floor, your lower back pressed into the floor. Either cross your arms across your chest or place your fingers lightly behind your ears. Slowly lift your upper body, bringing your shoulder blades off the floor 4 or 5 inches—*without* swinging your elbows forward. Now lower your shoulder blades to the floor, without letting your head touch the floor.

Three or four times a week, do as many crunches as you can without causing sharp or lingering pain. For most beginners, that's only 3 to 5. Don't start out trying for 25 or 50. In time, you should see an improvement in abdominal strength and back pain.

## BACK PAIN BOWS TO SOME BASICS

Despite millions of years on earth, humans are the product of their primitive genes; our bodies still respond best to the types of activities that kept muscles and bones supple and strong before the dawn of history. "All types of aerobic exercise stretch muscles and ligaments, but swimming and walking are among the best," says Dr. Nagler. It's also important to watch how you carry yourself and even how you sit.

**Try swimming or water aerobics.** With water to buoy the body, a simple swimming routine is still one of the best ways to treat back pain. "Swimming will relieve the stress on the lower back," says Dr. Nagler. If you don't like to swim—or can't—there are many beneficial water exercises you can do. (See chapter 1.)

**Get out and walk.** As long as posture is good, walking is also helpful. Posture is one of the keys to walking and sitting to benefit your back. "The adage that you should walk as if you had a book on your head is still the best advice you can receive for walking posture," says Dr. Faye. Don't lean forward while you walk; keep your head erect and straight. Also, keep your weight distributed from the middle of your feet forward, not on the back of your heels. "You want to walk so that you could stand up on your tiptoes, without rocking forward from your heels," says Dr. Faye.

**Support your lower back.** "Make sure that when you sit, there's a hollow in the small of your back," Dr. Faye suggests. Don't slouch while you're sitting. Keep your shoulders back, and tuck a rolled-up towel or small pillow between the base of your spine and the back of your chair.

## QUICK FIXES FOR FLARE-UPS

Here's what to do for nagging back pain.

**Get off your feet.** If pain doesn't go away after a day or two of taking it easy, head directly for bed for a couple of days, says Augustus A. White III, M.D., professor of orthopedic surgery at Harvard Medical School. Once the acute pain had passed, it's best to move around.

**Reach for an OTC.** If you feel you need medication for pain, aspirin is still the best bet, Dr. White says. Aspirin treats both the pain and the inflammation that causes the pain, as does ibuprofen. If you can't tolerate aspirin, take acetaminophen, which relieves pain but doesn't work on inflammation.

**Alternate ice and heat.** Meanwhile, alternately apply ice and moist heat, but limit the application of either to 20 minutes or less at a time. Ice will bring down the inflammation and may work better than heat during the first 48 hours after the injury, says Dr. White. Heat will stimulate blood flow and healing in the area.

## LITTLE THINGS CAN MEAN A LOT

Don't wait for full-blown pain to remind you that your back needs some TLC. As you go about your daily business, pay attention to the little things that really matter.

**Consider your shoes.** High heels or shoes that offer little or no support place excessive stress on the spine and especially the lower back, according to Dean Wakefield, director of public affairs at the American Podiatric Medical Association in Bethesda, Maryland.

**Bring breathing into the picture.** When stress, negative thinking and pain arise, breathe deeply, slowly and rhythmically. Back-care specialist Mike Hage says that breathing can help reduce discomfort and tension in the muscles.

**Get all the support you need in bed.** Does your pillow or mattress provide enough support? Either can increase muscle tension if it does not support the body during sleep. Check with an orthopedic specialist to help you select from a wide variety of pillows and mattresses that may offer you the improved rest and comfort that can make the difference.

**Stabilize your life.** "There is no single answer to back problems," says Dr. Faye. "You have to learn to balance your life in many ways, and that means a holistic approach in which the body and mind are related."

## ANTI-AGING CHECKUP
# THE HEALTHY BACK QUESTIONNAIRE

This will help you determine the extent of your back injury and whether you should see a physician, chiropractor or other back expert before beginning an exercise routine. Answer these questions Yes or No.

_____ Do you have constant back pain that is only relieved by aspirin or other painkillers?

_____ Is your constant pain or ache accompanied by great fatigue, the loss of appetite, weight loss or the need to urinate more frequently than usual?

_____ Does your back pain radiate through your genitals or affect your sex drive or your ability to urinate or become sexually aroused?

_____ If you have pain in one leg, sit on a chair and raise the good leg so that it's parallel with the floor. Do you feel pain in either your lower back or your bad leg?

_____ Has your back pain persisted constantly for more than a year?

_____ Do you have numbness in either of your thighs?

_____ Do you have difficulty walking on your toes or heels?

_____ Do you have severe leg pain without back pain?

## INTERPRETING YOUR ANSWERS

Answering Yes to any of these questions means that you should see a doctor, physical therapist or other health professional, says chiropractor Leonard Faye, D.C., author of *Good-Bye Back Pain!*

SOURCE: Adapted from *Good-Bye Back Pain!* by Leonard Faye, D.C. Copyright © 1990 by Leonard Faye, D.C. Reprinted by permission of Tale Weaver Publishing.

# 5

# BLADDER PROBLEMS

A Nuisance You *Don't* Have to Live With

**Bladder** trouble is rarely life-threatening, it's true. But it's one of those ailments that has a remarkable knack for making us feel miserable and out of control.

This is especially true for problems like urinary incontinence, the involuntary release of small amounts of urine. Understandably, this creates worry about going out in public for any length of time. Even though protective undergarments can help avoid embarrassing incidents, many people become reclusive because of their incontinence. They give up exercise, turn down certain kinds of job assignments (like travel), even avoid sex.

Many people plagued by bladder problems are too embarrassed or disheartened to seek help. But most bladder woes are curable or at least manageable. Here's what you can do to bring these conditions under control.

## BLADDERS CAN MISBEHAVE AT ANY AGE

Incontinence is commonly associated with growing older, but bladder problems are *not* a normal result of getting on in years. Nor is this disorder limited to senior citizens—both young and old can have bouts of incontinence, and middle-aged women are the most susceptible.

Incontinence can be triggered by a number of physical problems. These include urinary tract infections, constipation, weakness of the muscles that support the bladder and weakness of the sphincter muscle that controls the opening and closing of the urethra (the tube that carries urine from the bladder and out of the body). Other less common causes include overactive or underactive bladder muscles, neurological disorders, hormone imbalances in women and the effect of certain medications. Some studies suggest that people who are overweight may be predisposed to incontinence.

A common related disorder, cystitis, or inflammation of the urinary bladder, is often caused by bacterial infections. It can result in localized discomfort, pain when urinating and incontinence.

There are four basic types of incontinence.

**Stress incontinence.** Releasing small amounts of urine when laughing, sneezing, coughing or exercising often occurs among women who have given birth or postmenopausal women who have lost the beneficial effects of estrogen in maintaining muscle tone. During childbirth, the urethra may slip slightly from its normal position, so it can no longer close tightly enough to restrain the urine flow during movements that cause increased pressure on the bladder. After menopause, pelvic floor muscles that assist in the closure of the bladder outflow tract may atrophy, allowing urine to leak.

**Overflow incontinence.** Some people find they can no longer empty their bladder completely. They may leak small amounts of urine during the day and night but not be able to urinate when they try.

**Urge incontinence.** This kicks in when bladder nerves become unstable or hypersensitive. The person often feels a powerful need to urinate; sometimes it's impossible to get to the bathroom in time. A small drink of water or even the sound of running water can stimulate people with urge incontinence to urinate.

**Reflex incontinence.** With this disconcerting disorder, the person does not feel the urge to urinate, but the bladder empties anyway and without warning. This may be an indication of a serious neurological disorder, spinal cord compression or damage from diabetes, and it requires immediate medical evaluation.

### Exercise for Better Control

You can often train your bladder to behave by doing one or both of the exercises below. They are designed to restore control by increasing your sensitivity to your pelvic muscles, strengthening those muscles and making them more responsive to your commands.

**Do the bladder drill.** This technique requires that you urinate only at scheduled times during the day, usually one to two hours apart. Then, over a few weeks, gradually extend the periods between urinations—with a goal of reaching 2½ hours, then 3 hours.

Physicians recommend that you empty your bladder as completely as you can at your scheduled time, regardless of whether you feel an urge to go. If you feel an urgency to go again before your next scheduled trip to the toilet, try to distract yourself with work or some pleasant activity. If the urge becomes too great to be suppressed, of course you should go—*after* you have made a significant effort to resist.

Though it may take up to six months to regain the desired amount of control, this method of bladder training has been shown to be highly effective against incontinence, particularly for women with reflex incontinence. But both men and women can benefit.

**Perform Kegels daily.** Pelvic muscle exercise, also known as Kegel or postpartum exercise, has been used as an effective treatment for incontinence for more than a century. It calls for stopping and starting the flow of urine several times every time the bladder is being voided. Like any muscle-training regimen, these exercises must be done correctly and daily to have sustained benefits. Here is the proper technique.

1. Locate the proper muscles by placing your hands on your thighs and buttocks as you stop and start the urine flow. If these are tensed, you're doing the Kegels wrong. Focus instead on closing and opening the muscles that control the urethra and anus, which are the ones you want to strengthen.

2. Tighten the muscles slowly to the maximum extent you can; hold the contraction for 10 seconds; slowly release.
3. Repeat this exercise at least 10 times throughout the day.

As these muscles become stronger and larger, they work more efficiently, and you gain greater control over your bladder. Kegel exercises have proven remarkably successful against incontinence, with a cure rate of greater than 60 percent.

## HELP YOUR BLADDER BEHAVE

Besides performing Kegels and bladder drills, there are other steps you can take to prevent "accidents." Here are a few.

**Hit the john before you hit the track.** Women who perform high-impact aerobics tend to report frequent loss of bladder control, according to a study done by John Delancey, M.D., at the University of Michigan. After studying 326 women ages 17 to 68, he found that more than a third of those who ran or did high-impact aerobics had bladder-control problems during their workouts.

Dr. Delancey advises emptying the bladder before exercise and doing Kegels daily. If the problem persists, he suggests switching to a more bladder-friendly regimen, such as bicycle riding.

**Eliminate the irritants.** Diet can play a role in incontinence, according to the *Public Citizen Health Research Group Health Letter*. Studies have shown that caffeine, alcohol, sugar, acidic juices and foods, spicy foods and milk products can irritate the bladder, causing hypersensitivity and urge incontinence. Try eliminating such foods from your diet to see if that has any effect on your bladder control. Also, chronic alcohol abuse can severely weaken the bladder muscle, resulting in overflow incontinence.

**Quit smoking.** Research at the Medical College of Virginia at Richmond suggests that about one-third of all women suffering from urinary incontinence may be able to trace the cause of their problem to present or past smoking. The scientists found that smokers and former smokers experience twice the risk of all types of incontinence, compared with nonsmokers. The problem, say some doctors, may be that violent coughing caused by smoking weakens bladder muscles or that nicotine causes the muscles to contract.

**Take off pounds of pressure.** If you are overweight and suffering from incontinence, the best thing to do is shed some of those unwanted pounds to take some of the strain off your bladder and pelvic muscles. A study in the *Journal of Urology* reported that body mass was directly associated with higher rates of incontinence. Researcher Kathryn L. Burgio and her colleagues concluded that weight gain may increase susceptibility to incontinence and that weight loss may help solve the problem. (For pound-paring tips, see chapter 27.)

**Monitor your fluids.** Caffeine-containing beverages act as diuretics, so pass them up, says Maria Fiatarone, M.D., chief of the physiology laboratory at the U.S. Department of Agriculture's Human Nutrition Research Center on Aging at Tufts University in Boston and assistant professor in the division on aging at Harvard Medical School. This includes coffee, tea, cocoa and some sodas (check labels). Likewise, give up alcohol, which can also act as a diuretic. And if nighttime incontinence is a problem, stop drinking fluids after 6:00 P.M. (Urinate just before bedtime.)

**Improve voiding technique.** You can empty your bladder more completely by pressing on it (just above the pubic bone) while bending forward at the waist, says Dr. Fiatarone. This is helpful when the bladder muscle is weak or when the prostate gland is enlarged.

**Seek professional help.** If self-help techniques don't help, see your doctor. There may be a drug or medical condition causing your incontinence. Also, a number of medications are available to treat incontinence. "Above all, do not resign yourself to wearing pads or adult diapers the rest of your life, as most causes of incontinence are remediable if not completely curable," says Dr. Fiatarone.

### A SIMPLE SYSTEM TO FIGHT CYSTITIS

Cystitis—an inflammation of the urinary bladder that's commonly due to bacterial infection of the urinary tract—causes burning and pain during urination. It also causes a strong urge to urinate, plus incontinence, blood in the urine and sometimes soreness in the lower abdomen or back.

In women, cystitis is second only to colds in frequency. The reason it's so common is that it's a relatively short journey for the bacteria *Escherichia coli* to migrate from the rectum to the vagina, then up the urethra and into the bladder. (*E. coli* infections are considered the primary culprit of cystitis.) They can be treated with antibiotics, but it's preferable to *avoid* the problem. Here's what you can do.

**Keep the system well flushed.** To prevent urinary tract infection, drink ample amounts of water—six to eight 8-ounce glasses a day, say doctors. Water helps flush bacteria out of your bladder.

**Wipe front to back.** After using the bathroom, *don't* wipe from back to front, which could push bacteria from the rectum toward the urethra, says Joshua Hoffman, M.D., an internist in private practice in Sacramento, California. Always wipe the rectal area toward the back, he says.

**Urinate after sex.** There are always bacteria around the vagina, and sexual intercourse can contribute to cystitis by pushing bacteria toward the urethra. Emptying the bladder after sex will help to flush out any wayward bacteria, says Dr. Hoffman.

**Reconsider the diaphragm.** In some cases, women who use diaphragms for birth control are plagued by bladder infections, possibly because the insertion and removal of the device give bacteria a chance for a free ride. If you're having bladder problems, consider using another method of birth control.

**ANTI-AGING CHECKUP**
# 12 SIGNS OF A WEAK BLADDER

Answer the following questions Yes or No to help you determine whether you have incontinence (and if you do, what kind).

**URGE INCONTINENCE**

_____ Do you frequently feel such an overwhelming need to urinate that you cannot get to the bathroom quickly enough?

_____ When you hear water running or when you drink even a sip of water, do you feel a powerful urge to urinate?

_____ Do you have to urinate as frequently as once very two hours?

_____ Is the urge to urinate so strong that it often causes you to leak?

**STRESS INCONTINENCE**

_____ Do you leak urine when you sneeze, cough or laugh?

_____ Do you leak urine when you rise from a chair or bed?

_____ Does exercise or walking cause leaking?

**OVERFLOW INCONTINENCE**

_____ Are you unable to empty your bladder completely?

_____ Do you lose small amounts of urine during the day or night?

_____ Are you up often during the night to urinate?

_____ Do you frequently feel the urge to empty your bladder but find that you can't?

_____ Do you pass only a small amount of urine but feel that your bladder is still full?

_____ In spite of spending a long time trying to void, do you produce only a weak, dribbling stream of urine?

**INTERPRETING YOUR ANSWERS**

If your bladder isn't performing up to par, don't suffer in silence: Try the self-help tips outlined in this chapter. If they don't help, see your doctor.

# 6

# BLOOD PRESSURE

### Don't Let It Sneak Up on You

**High** blood pressure is sneaky: Symptoms can be subtle and easily overlooked. Few people would ever know they had high blood pressure (hypertension) unless a doctor spotted it in a routine checkup.

Left untreated, hypertension dramatically increases your chances of suffering a stroke or heart attack or dying of congestive heart failure. It can also contribute to kidney disease and problems with eyesight. Experts say that the simple and painless act of having a blood pressure reading taken regularly could save 15,000 lives *every* year.

So if your vision of the future is based on a long and problem-free life, get your blood pressure checked, if you haven't already, and take steps to lower it. But first, here's a little information to set the stage for action.

### BLOOD PRESSURE POSES FOR A PROFILE

Your blood pressure reading simply reflects the effort your heart puts into pushing the blood through your main arteries. The pressure rises as the heart beats faster when you exercise or face stress, and it falls as the heart beats more slowly when you sit or sleep.

Blood pressure is expressed as a fraction—for example, 110/75 (a healthy reading for a young adult). The top number indicates the pressure created when the heart contracts, called the systolic phase. The bottom number represents the pressure between beats, called the diastolic phase, and measures the resistance of the small arteries.

Blood pressure is expressed as millimeters of mercury (mm Hg), which harks back to early blood pressure gauges that measured pressure by how high mercury was raised in a calibrated tube. Today, the gauge—called a sphygmomanometer or a blood pressure cuff—uses a spring, and a reading takes only a few minutes.

Blood pressure readings rise with age in the United States, although not in some less industrialized nations. Healthy blood pressure for most people is 130/90 at age 60, while any reading that consistently hits 140/90 or higher is considered risky. Notice the word *consistently*. Your blood pressure fluctuates throughout the day with your activity and stress levels, which is perfectly normal. The real problems arise when it increases and *stays* elevated.

Many people also experience a temporary rise in blood pressure the moment they walk into a doctor's office. "If someone shows a high blood pressure on the first visit with me and there aren't a lot of other risk factors, such as being overweight or smoking, I check the pressure over several visits before I do anything about it," says Charles Tifft, M.D., associate professor of medicine at Boston University School of Medicine. "What you find is that a lot of people have temporarily high pressure that 'washes out,' or normalizes, after they begin to relax."

## TUNE IN TO AN EXERCISE PROGRAM

Regular aerobic exercise can prevent hypertension or lower existing high blood pressure. Many people are able to cut back on blood pressure medication (or do without it entirely) simply by adopting a regular exercise program. Any aerobic exercise will do the job, but walking is the safest.

"You don't need to walk far or long, and you shouldn't at first," says Paul D. Thompson, M.D., director of the Cardiovascular Disease Prevention Center at the University of Pittsburgh Heart Institute. "You need to walk a minimum of 30 minutes, three to five times a week."

One caveat: If you're taking medication for high blood pressure, talk to your doctor before starting an exercise program. Keep him or her informed of your progress, and don't discontinue or cut back on your medication unless your physician says you should.

### SHAKE THE SALT HABIT

For half of those with high blood pressure, sodium is a major cause. Salt, which is about 40 percent sodium, is the prime source of excess dietary sodium.

Actually, the body requires some salt—about one-fourth teaspoon per day—to maintain normal blood pressure as well as healthy nerve and muscle function, says George Blackburn, M.D., Ph.D., chief of the nutrition/metabolism laboratory at New England Deaconess Hospital in Boston and associate professor of medicine at Harvard Medical School. But you can easily get that amount from a diet rich in fruit, grains, vegetables and fish or poultry—with *no* added salt. The National Academy of Sciences recommends that healthy people eat no more than 1½ teaspoons of salt per day. Dr. Blackburn suggests the following ways to stay within your salt-intake limit.

**Cook salt-free.** In the vast majority of dishes, you can skip the salt entirely. And you don't need to add it when boiling pasta. Use reduced amounts for certain dishes, such as chicken soup or homemade bread (to control yeast action).

**Season your food creatively.** Use vinegars, lemon and lime juice, herbs and spices as flavorings. Cook with liberal quantities of chopped onions, garlic, basil and oregano. Make your own salt-free herb blends.

**Scrutinize labels.** All processed foods marked "low sodium" contain no more than 140 milligrams of sodium per serving. "Very low sodium" products must contain 35 milligrams or less. One catch: Serving sizes listed for chips, salad dressings and so forth tend to be small. You may be regularly consuming more than what's considered one helping, so check the serving size as well.

## Four Powerful Hypertension Fighters

Okay, you've cut back on salt and increased your exercise. Yes, there's still more you can easily do to help reduce blood pressure levels.

**Take a vacation from alcohol intake.** While a drink or two may lower blood pressure, higher amounts elevate it. If alcohol is part of your life, consider cutting down. And if you drink every day, think about giving it a rest for at least a few days (or nights) a week. A study in the *American Journal of Pubic Health* compared people who drank daily with those who drank once a week. The daily imbibers had systolic pressures that averaged 6.6 mm Hg higher and diastolic pressures of 4.7 mm Hg higher than those who drank once a week.

**Toss the cigarettes.** Smoking a single cigarette raises blood pressure for 30 minutes to an hour. That means a pack-a-day habit can keep blood pressure elevated all day, every day. Smoking also raises LDL cholesterol and causes antherosclerosis.

**Trim down.** Numerous studies show that one of the most powerful tools for lowering blood pressure is losing excess weight. In one study of hypertensive people, 60 percent of those who lost weight normalized their blood pressure *without* medication.

While excess weight alone is enough to raise blood pressure, losing belly fat may be especially crucial. A report in the journal *Hypertension* found that overweight women with prominent pot-bellies had higher blood pressure than women whose pounds were more evenly distributed.

**Combine strategies.** "In general, the best approach to prevent and control moderately high blood pressure is one that involves multiple lifestyle factors, including healthy diet, weight control and exercise," says Dr. Blackburn.

A combined program of exercise, weight loss and salt reduction allowed people ages 60 to 85 with mildly high blood pressure to eliminate medication, researcher William B. Applegate, M.D., and colleagues reported in *Archives of Internal Medicine*. Those folks exercised four times a week, 30 minutes a session.

When researchers in England investigated which of three

dietary strategies worked best against hypertension—eating less fat, less sodium or more fiber—they found that no one approach worked as well as combining all three.

### A Diet to Knock Down Blood Pressure

"Elevated blood cholesterol levels are associated with greater risk of high blood pressure," says Dr. Tifft. The cholesterol-lowering tips that follow relate directly to blood pressure.

**Minimize fat, maximize fiber.** Research consistently shows that vegetarians as a group have lower blood pressure and are less likely to become hypertensive than nonvegetarians. Simply by reducing the saturated fat and increasing the fiber in your diet, you can lower your blood pressure. In general, meats and dairy products are high in saturated fats, and fiber-rich choices include whole grains and most fruits and vegetables. (For details, see chapters 8 and 19.)

**Pump up your potassium intake.** A study reported in the *Annals of Internal Medicine* showed that eating potassium-rich foods, such as fruit, vegetables and grains, lowered blood pressure in 12 hypertensive people. But when potassium-containing foods were withheld, their blood pressure rose significantly. When a large amount of salt was added to the low-potassium diet, blood pressure rose even more sharply.

"A low-potassium intake may substantially increase your risk of getting hypertension or, we now suspect, may make the existing high blood pressure worse," says researcher G. Gopal Krishna, M.D., associate professor of medicine at the University of Pennsylvania in Philadelphia. "Studies in animals and humans suggest, though, that when you get the right amount of potassium, the positive change in blood pressure may lead to a reduction in risk of stroke." So concentrate on such potassium bonanzas as bananas, potatoes, broccoli, tomatoes and orange juice.

**Consider the calcium factor.** Some studies have suggested that as calcium intake increases, blood pressure drops—especially if you're low in calcium to start with. And a study reported in the *New England Journal of Medicine* found that pregnant women who received calcium supplements developed fewer problems associated with high blood pressure than women who didn't get the supplements. Healthy sources of calcium include low-fat milk, cheese and yogurt, and sardines and salmon if you eat the bones.

## HOSTILITY IS A BOOMERANG

Everyone gets angry, depressed or stressed out sometimes, but how you behave in these situations can make all the difference to your blood pressure.

**Fight nicely.** In a study published in *Health Psychology,* Johns Hopkins researcher Craig Ewart, Ph.D., and his colleagues examined the effects arguments had on couples with hypertension. As might be expected, the marital disagreements led to elevated blood pressures in both men and women, but for different reasons. The men's blood pressure rose whey they spoke faster and louder, while the women's jumped during hostile interactions and when feelings of marital dissatisfaction surfaced.

Behavior likely to cause hikes in blood pressure included attacking the other person verbally, impugning his or her motives, refusing to listen or making excuses. Dr. Ewart suggests that when partners argue, they should phrase their disagreements in ways that focus on how *they* feel, rather than accusing or blaming the other person. For example, say "When you make jokes about my mother, it makes me very unhappy," rather than "You are so rude to joke about my mother." This approach gets the point across without directly attacking the other person.

Men especially should avoid talking rapidly and loudly because that tends to elevate their blood pressure and that of their partners.

**Learn to relax.** A smart move to take when you feel tense or depressed is to induce the "relaxation response," a physiologically relaxed condition made possible by choosing to concentrate on peaceful images or words, says Herbert Benson, M.D., associate professor of medicine at Harvard Medical School.

Sit quietly in a comfortable position; close your eyes and empty your mind. Breathe deeply and rhythmically. Concentrate on a single word or phrase that is not related to the immediate situation. Gradually, anxiety, tension, depression and anger will fade. "These emotions are related to rises in blood pressure," says Dr. Benson.

Such stress-management techniques have reduced mild hypertension and effectively counteracted increases in blood pressure when patients were taken off medication. "Meditation, progressive muscular relaxation and short prayer are all ways to elicit this response," Dr. Benson says. "The key is to find one method you're comfortable with and stick with it."

---

**ANTI-AGING CHECKUP**
# TAKE YOUR BLOOD PRESSURE AT HOME

Blood pressure cuffs, or sphygmomanometers, that are both inexpensive and accurate can be purchased at most pharmacies or medical-supply stores. Your doctor or pharmacist can advise you on the type best suited for you and how to use the device. Then compare the accuracy of the device against your doctor's reading.

Not sure about the accuracy of your readings? Answer these questions Yes or No.

_____ Is the cuff too small to accommodate your arm?
_____ Was your bladder full when the reading was taken?
_____ Were you lying down, rather than standing or sitting?
_____ Did you take multiple readings without waiting one minute between each reading?
_____ Were you tensing your arm muscles during the reading?

## INTERPRETING YOUR ANSWERS

If the answer to any of these questions was Yes, your result is dubious. Try again.

If you get consistently *lower* readings at home, your elevated readings at the doctor's office may be because of "white coat hypertension," blood pressure that zooms at the sight of a doctor. If you or your doctor suspect this is the case, consider having a nurse take your blood pressure—studies show that blood pressure readings tend to be lower when taken by a nurse.

# 7

# BURSITIS

## What to Do When Pain Strikes

**Despite** its quaint nicknames—housemaid's knee, student's elbow and clergyman's knee—bursitis is no laughing matter.

This painful condition occurs when your bursae, the tiny fluid-filled sacs that serve as cushions in and around the joints, become swollen. The most common cause is overuse of certain joints, especially in activities that are out of the ordinary for you. This could be taking on your teenager in yet another round of one-on-one basketball, painting the kitchen or playing too many sets of tennis. As bursae rub against muscles, tendons and each other, they become irritated, swollen and painful.

Bursitis can also be caused by pressure—hence those descriptive nicknames. Kneeling to scrub a floor or roof a house puts pressure on the bursae of the knee, for example. A shoe that's too tight can cause a swollen bursa, called a pump bump.

Most commonly, bursitis strikes the shoulders, says Patrick Guiteras, M.D., clinical faculty member at the University of North Carolina at Chapel Hill School of Medicine. Other common sites are the elbows, hips and knees. Fortunately, the condition usually passes within a few days to a week or two.

### DOUSE THE FIRE

When bursitis hits, the first thing to do is stop the activity that caused the problem. Then attend to pain with the following treatments.

**Chill it.** Immediately apply an ice pack or ice wrapped in a towel to the trouble joint to bring down the swelling. Leave it on for ten minutes, several times a day.

**Apply moist heat.** After the swelling has disappeared, warm up the area by taking a shower or bath, apply hot towels or relaxing in a heated whirlpool. Heat increases blood circulation to the affected area, which helps it heal.

**Take an OTC.** An over-the-counter medication such as aspirin or ibuprofen will help reduce swelling and pain. Check with your doctor first if you have a history of stomach ulcers or irritation.

**Keep moving.** Although you don't want to repeat the activity that *caused* the bursitis, it's important that you don't stop moving, particularly if your shoulders are injured. Otherwise, the joint will become stiff and can "freeze."

**Eliminate the pressure.** Try to keep pressure off the affected area. If the bursitis is in your shoulder or elbow, for example, try to sleep on your back or on the side opposite that joint.

### LOOSEN AFFECTED JOINTS THROUGH EXERCISE

As the pain and swelling decrease, begin doing any of the exercises described below. (For knee and leg exercises, see chapter 21.) Consult your doctor before doing any strenuous chore or exercise. If you get the go-ahead, be sure to warm up by stretching muscles and tendons before you start the workout. This will make the muscles and tendons more flexible and limber so they won't press so hard on the bursae. Do these exercises three times a day.

**Touch your elbows.** Clasp your hands behind your head. Now bring your elbows together in front of your face, as close as possible to one another. Then separate them as widely as you can. Repeat, gradually working up to 10 repetitions.

**Reach out.** Stretch one arm straight out in front of you.

Lock your elbow, and raise your arm directly over your head so that your fingers are pointing toward the ceiling. Lower the arm. Do 5 to 10 repetitions for each arm.

**Rotate your arms.** Stretch one arm out from your side so that it is parallel with the floor. Now rotate that arm in small circles forward, then in reverse. Work your way up from 5 to 10 circles, then 20, in both directions. Repeat with the other arm.

**Reach for the stars.** Raise your arms above and behind your head as far as possible. Do not force the motion; just try to gradually improve the distance you can reach backward. Do 5, then 10, then 20 repetitions. (If your arms hurt or you have trouble raising them, try lying on your bed and holding a broom handle or some other stick in both hands to help you stretch.)

**Roll your shoulders.** Begin by raising your shoulders toward your ears, then roll them back so that your chest sticks out. Next, roll them down, then forward and up. Work your way up from 5 repetitions to 10, then 20.

**Do shoulder touches.** Extend one arm directly out at your side, parallel with the floor. Touch your shoulder with your hand by bending at the elbow and bringing your hand back to the top of your shoulder. Work your way up from 5 repetitions to 10, then 20. Repeat with the other arm.

**Lift your leg.** While lying on a firm mat or on your bed, lift one leg, knee bent, and bring it toward your chest. You can use your hands to grab hold below your thigh. Do 5, 10 or 20 repetitions per leg.

## SOLVE THE PROBLEM

You can keep some cases of bursitis from recurring. Here's how.

**Change your shoes.** If your bursitis is caused by shoes that are too tight in the heel, try a heel lift. If that doesn't work, you may have to ditch the shoes. If they're too tight in the toes, either get rid of them or see if they can be stretched enough to solve the problem.

**Analyze your stroke.** Bursitis in swimmers' shoulders, the result of muscle imbalance or overuse, can be caused by either rolling too much as you swim or not rolling enough with each stroke. Ask a swim coach or instructor to analyze your stroke; better yet, have it videotaped so you can pinpoint the problem on your own.

**Add a pad.** Bursitis caused by constant kneeling or sitting is easily prevented: Carry a cushion or pad with you to sit or kneel on. This will reduce the pressure on your joints.

**Switch chores around.** Because repetitive motion causes bursae to become inflamed, you can sometimes circumvent the problem by alternating chores. Don't spend a whole day painting the kitchen or raking the yard; enlist help, or break up the job into two-hour segments.

# 8

# CHOLESTEROL

## Scour This Goo from Your Arteries

**Your** cholesterol reading may be a better indicator of your state of health than the number of birthdays you've had. The amount of cholesterol in your blood can help predict your chances of having a heart attack or stroke, and that tells you a lot about the number of years you can expect are ahead of you.

For example, in populations such as the Chinese that ordinarily consume low-fat, low-cholesterol diets, the rates of both cardiovascular disease and many common cancers are relatively low. But when changes in diet cause a hike in cholesterol levels among these people, the rates of heart attack and stroke climb as well.

The lesson is clear. The lower your cholesterol levels, the higher your chances for good health.

### BREAKING THE CHOLESTEROL CODE

First, let's take a look at what your cholesterol reading means and how it stacks up against recommended healthy levels. Say you just received the results of your cholesterol test; the reading is 225 mg/dl (milligrams per deciliter of blood). "No real cause for alarm; we'll just keep an eye on it," says your doctor. What does she mean?

**Understand the numbers.** Experts generally advise that you keep your total cholesterol level below 200 mg/dl. According to Abbey Ershow, Sc.D., a nutrition researcher at the National Heart, Lung and Blood Institute, a reading of 200 to

239 is considered borderline, and anything above 239 is considered high risk for heart attack or stroke.

The consensus among most researchers and physicians is that a person whose total cholesterol level is 200 mg/dl needn't be checked for a change more than once every five years. However, a person whose level falls between 200 and 240 should be checked yearly.

**Consider trying for a lower level.** More conservative researchers argue for lowering the so-called safe levels to 160 or 150 mg/dl as a protective measure against cardiovascular disease. "About four billion people on this earth have a cholesterol level of 150. And they don't get cardiovascular disease," says William Castelli, M.D., director of the Framingham Heart Study, a long-term study gathering health-related data on the adult residents of Framingham, Massachusetts. "If we pushed our cholesterol more toward this level, we could share in some of the good fortune of those four billion people."

**Meet the good and bad cholesterols.** Much depends on the two types of fat or lipoproteins that make up the total cholesterol level figure. LDL (low density lipoprotein) is sometimes called the bad cholesterol, and HDL (high density lipoprotein) is known as the good cholesterol. High levels of LDL can cause atherosclerosis, or clogging of the arteries that transport blood to the heart, brain and other organs. High levels of *HDL,* however, protect against this clogging by helping to transport LDL out of the body.

**Beware of triglycerides.** Triglycerides are the fatty acids that migrate into the bloodstream when we consume foods rich in fat and sugar. Some scientists believe triglycerides cause the blood to thicken into sludge, reducing blood flow to the heart and other organs. A triglyceride level considered desirable is 150mg/dl. To keep your level low, cut your consumption of fatty or sweet foods, avoid excessive alcohol, and maintain a normal body weight. If you have diabetes, keep it under good control with diet, exercise or medications prescribed by your doctor.

## 11 Easy Steps to Reduce Cholesterol Levels

So you've gotten your cholesterol measured, and you need to bring it down. Here are some of the best cholesterol-cutting measures you can take.

**Cut meat intake.** Most Americans get 13 percent of their total calories from saturated fat. Cardiologists would like to see that figure drop to about 7 percent. To that end, limit lean meat, poultry or fish to a 3-ounce portion (about the size of a deck of cards) no more than once a day. Only animal foods contain cholesterol and saturated fat. Therefore, the foods that drive up your blood cholesterol numbers most are red meats, the skin of poultry, whole dairy products and eggs. Fish, especially the white-fleshed ones, tend to be low in saturated fat.

**Take a holiday from the fat flow.** To make sure your cholesterol level goes down, cut *all* fat intake—including vegetable oils—to 25 percent or, even better, 20 percent of total calories. That will guarantee less saturated fat consumption. Here are ways to accomplish this.

- Eat red meat no more than two or three times per week.
- Eat at least two meatless meals a day.
- Choose fat-free condiments, such as mustard, horseradish, nonfat salad dressings, catsup, chili sauce, relish and salsa, rather than fatty ones such as mayonnaise or regular salad dressing.

**Go vegetarian.** If your high cholesterol just won't go down even though you've cut back on fat, go on a vegetarian diet of whole grains, fresh vegetables, beans, fruit and a limited amount of low-fat dairy products. Dean Ornish, M.D., director of the Preventive Medicine Research Institute in Sausalito, California, and author of *Dr. Dean Ornish's Program for Reversing Heart Disease,* has shown that a vegetarian diet, coupled with exercise and meditation, can dramatically lower blood cholesterol levels and reverse the atherosclerostic plaques that form the basis for heart disease.

**Feast on high fiber.** If you're overweight *and* have high cholesterol, increasing your fiber intake to 20 to 35 grams of fiber each day may help lower cholesterol. (Most of us eat 10 grams or less a day.) Chow down on foods such as oats, brown rice, whole-grain products, legumes, apples and citrus fruits. The soluble fiber in oats and psyllium seeds are particularly effective in lowering cholesterol.

At Central Washington University in Ellensburg, researchers studied 26 men with blood cholesterol in the 200- to 250-mg/dl range. Thirteen of the men added fiber-rich apple cookies to the diets daily for six weeks. Final blood tests showed that the cholesterol level of the apple-fiber group was lowered by an average of 15 mg/dl, or about 7 percent, with no other dietary changes.

Eating about 2 ounces of oat bran (a medium-size bowl) or 3 ounces of oatmeal (a large bowl) once a day, in addition to eating a low-fat, low cholesterol diet, can lower LDL cholesterol (the bad kind) 10 to 15 percent, concluded Michael H. Davidson, M.D., medical director of the Chicago Center for Clinical Research and assistant professor at Rush Presbyterian–St. Luke's Medical Center, after observing 148 adults with high cholesterol levels.

**Ease into the "good" oils.** Choose monounsaturated or polyunsaturated oils from nuts and grains rather than saturated fats from animal sources. Olive oil is your best bet, but other good options include canola, safflower, corn and sunflower oils. Other less common choices are barley oil and amaranth oil. In a study by Joanne Lupton, Ph.D., chair of the graduate faculty in nutrition at Texas A&M University in College Station, the use of barley flour and barley oils reduced overall cholesterol by 7 percent and LDL by nearly 9.2 percent. Amaranth oils have a similar cholesterol-lowering effect. Remember that *all* forms of fat are laden with calories, however, and keep your intake of fat to a minimum.

**Fish for the superfats.** Almost all fish contain some omega-3 fatty acids, whose chemical makeup keeps these fats liquid even in very low temperatures (essential for cold-water fish). Omega-3s help lower blood fat levels and heart disease risk. They also help prevent the development of blood clots, which can severely restrict blood flow to the heart.

Certain fish are particularly rich in omega-3s and low in fat. A 3½-ounce serving of sea bass contains 595 milligrams of omega-3s and only 2 grams of fat; 3½ ounces of Atlantic pollack has 421 milligrams of omega-3s and just 1 gram of fat. Snapper and Pacific Rockfish are also very high in omega-3s and very low in total fat. Your efforts to cut down on fatty foods will get a big boost if you include low-fat, high-omega-3 fish in your diet.

**Combine exercise with weight loss.** If you take at least 30 minutes, three or four times a week, to enjoy an aerobic exercise such as walking, bicycling, swimming, tennis, running or golf, your heart will thank you. (For those with heart disease, walking is perhaps the safest aerobic exercise.)

For people who are overweight, aerobic exercise, when combined with weight loss, is known to lower total cholesterol levels and particularly LDLs. But more than that, it is one of the few things you can do to raise your HDL level. And you don't need to work all that hard to benefit. "A brisk walk 20 minutes a day would make a major impact," says Thomas Kottke, M.D., a cardiologist at the Mayo Clinic in Rochester, Minnesota.

Even the walking involved in playing a few rounds of golf each week may lower your LDLs, suggests a study by Edward A. Palank, M.D., director of the New Hampshire Heart Institute. He reported on 28 men with normal to mildly elevated cholesterol levels who golfed three times a week for four months. They averaged 14 miles of walking per week, while pulling a cart or carrying a light bag and avoiding the golf cart entirely. The result; "Their LDL cholesterol dropped significantly, while their HDL cholesterol stayed the same," says Dr. Palank. A group of 16 men who played no golf saw no improvement.

**Help your heart with vitamin C.** Foods rich in vitamin C help keep your HDL cholesterol levels up. And if your diet includes such C-rich items as broccoli, cabbage, citrus fruits and strawberries, you also benefit from fiber, which can help remove LDL cholesterol.

People who consume significant amounts of vitamin C regularly have higher HDLs, according to findings of the Baltimore Longitudinal Study of Aging. Among the 800 men and women (ages 20 to 95) tested, those with the highest blood levels of C had HDL levels that were approximately 5 mg/dl higher than those with the lowest levels of C.

**Puff no more.** Smoking raises your LDL and total cholesterol, increases the formation of cholesterol plaque and lowers HDLs. If you continue to smoke, you're twice as likely to have heart disease and a heart attack than nonsmokers. In 1989, smoking killed 115,000 people from heart disease (and 9,000 more from lung cancer).

The best advice is to avoid smoking if you haven't started and stop if you have. For help in quitting, ask your doctor how you can locate a stop-smoking group approved by the American Lung Association.

**Relax.** "Emotions play a powerful role in affecting your body and especially your heart," Dr. Ornish says. "I believe that it's not enough to ask people to change their behavior without also addressing the emotional factors that underlie the behaviors." He advises people to use relaxation techniques, including yoga, imaging routines and group therapy, to control stress and reduce cholesterol levels.

**Women, ask your doctor about HRT.** Estrogen helps control cholesterol, so levels can climb after menopause, when estrogen production falls dramatically. Hormone replacement therapy (HRT) which contains estrogen, can raise HDL and lower LDL toward premenopausal levels. Ask your doctor if you could benefit from such therapy. (HRT isn't recommended for everyone.)

**ANTI-AGING CHECKUP**
# HOW RISKY ARE YOUR CHOLESTEROL LEVELS?

The ratio of HDL to total cholesterol may well be the best predictor of heart attack yet discovered. In one study, blood samples of 246 men from the Physician's Heart Study who had had heart attacks were compared with samples of those who hadn't. According to a report in the *New England Journal of Medicine,* the standout risk factor was the ratio of total cholesterol to HDL cholesterol. Those with the highest ratios had nearly four times the risk as men with lower ratios.

To get your own ratio, divide your total cholesterol number by your HDL number. If your total cholesterol is 250 mg/dl and your HDL is 50, your ratio is 5:1. If you get your total cholesterol down to 200 and your HDL stays at 50, the ratio drops to 4:1 (200 divided by 50). Dropping your ratio one full point reduces your chance of having a heart attack by 53 percent.

A ratio of total cholesterol to HDL that is less than 3.5:1 puts you among the lucky ones who have little chance of getting heart disease, says William Castelli, M.D., director of the Framingham Heart Study, a long-term study gathering health-related data on the adult residents of Framingham, Massachusetts. You should still be careful to monitor your fatty food intake, however, and get plenty of exercise.

# 9

# CIRCULATION

Keep Circulatory Problems at Bay

**When** all the technical information about your circulatory system is boiled down to its simplest terms, two things are obvious: When circulation moves steadily and unhampered, that's good; when it doesn't, that's bad.

Techniques designed to "improve your circulation" simply try to help keep blood flowing at a rate and volume scientists consider normal. When the blood flow to tissues is too slow or is inadequate, cells suffocate for lack of oxygen, causing pain, numbness, cold fingers or toes, frequent bruising, infection or worse. Collectively, these conditions are signs of peripheral vascular disease (PVD).

The most common symptom of PVD is claudication due to atherosclerosis or cholesterol plaques that clog the arteries in the legs. But many people suffer from other vascular illnesses, including Raynaud's phenomenon and phlebitis, which have their own specific causes. Let's look at these ailments individually and see how they can be prevented or relieved.

### CLAUDICATION: PAIN THAT STOPS YOU IN YOUR TRACKS

More than five million Americans suffer from claudication, a disease that prevents them from walking more than a block or two without severe pain. Symptoms include painful cramping in the thighs and calves, usually after walking a very short distance. This pain can become severe enough to restrict a person to a wheelchair. Like many forms of heart disease, claudication is caused primarily by a high-fat, high-cholesterol diet and cigarette smoking.

Because atherosclerosis is the underlying illness, far more perilous side effects may occur. "The biggest concern people with claudication should have is their elevated risk of having a heart attack or stroke," says William B. Kannel, M.D., professor of medicine and public health and chief of preventive medicine and epidemiology at Boston University School of Medicine. "Claudication indicates that the person has diffuse vascular disease, which can affect the coronary arteries leading to their heart or the carotid artery leading to the brain." Indeed, studies show that about one out of every two people with claudication will die of a heart attack.

Claudication causes increased incidence of gangrene and amputations, resulting from insufficient circulation to the limbs. Lack of proper blood flow also means a deficiency of immune cells in the area, which translates into a higher rate of infections and ischemic (skin) ulcers that take a long time to heal, according to Dr. Kannel.

### SIX STRATEGIES TO BYPASS CLAUDICATION

Don't wait for trouble to seek you out. An objective self-evaluation will tell you what steps to take as insurance against circulation woes. Here are some ways to help avoid problems. (For more details, see individual chapters on each health problem mentioned.)

**Cut away the fat.** As explained in the chapters on heart disease and cholesterol, a low-fat, low-cholesterol diet has been shown to reverse the development of plaque that blocks the vessels in the first place.

**Bring down your blood pressure.** High blood pressure causes cracks and fissures in the protective inner lining of blood vessels, trapping atherosclerotic plaque.

**Control diabetes.** People with diabetes have a higher-than-average risk of suffering from claudication as well as many other forms of cardiovascular disease. They also have a much higher risk of amputation, blindness, heart disease and stroke due to artery blockage, says Dr. Kannel.

**Concentrate on foot care.** Keeping feet clean is a simple but often overlooked way for people with PVD to avoid infections, says Dr. Kannel. Keep toenails trimmed, avoid going barefoot, take action to heal cracks and ulcers of the feet, and see a podiatrist for regular checkups.

**Keep warm.** Cold temperatures cause blood vessels to constrict, diminishing blood flow. Those who live in cold climates should take special care to keep feet and hands well covered in winter to prevent frostbite and gangrene.

**Don't wear tight-fitting clothes.** Any garment that might limit blood flow can be dangerous in the presence of PVD. This applies especially to belts, garters or stockings that are tight at the bottom of the foot and looser at the top.

## How to Deal with Claudication

If you do suffer from claudication, there are many therapies available. Here are a few.

**Stop smoking.** "Many of the people who claudicate are smokers," says Dr. Kannel. Cigarette smoking raises LDL ("bad") cholesterol, lowers HDL ("good") cholesterol and promotes the formation of fat deposits in the arteries.

**Start walking.** Researchers at the University of Colorado School of Medicine studied the effects of walking on a group of people with claudication. All walked a total of one hour per day, and after 12 weeks the participants had doubled the amount of time they were able to walk without pain.

In another study, 14 people with claudication walked daily for one year, while a control group was given a placebo (a pill with no active ingredient). The exercisers increased their walking distance 300 percent, on average, while the placebo group showed no significant improvement.

Exercise not only reduces the pain, it also improves the efficiency with which muscles absorb and utilize oxygen. This occurs in several ways. Many small blood vessels that would remain closed under sedentary conditions open up when muscles demand greater quantities of blood and oxygen during exercise. A study published in the *American Journal of Cardiology* demonstrated that this also occurs in the coronary arteries, the vessels that provide blood and oxygen to the heart.

Other researchers report that regular exercise may even trigger growth of new blood vessels to meet the increased demands for oxygen. Consequently, tissues receive oxygen from secondary vessels (also known as collaterals) and from newly created vessels, which compensate for the blocked arteries. By improving blood flow, exercise also floods areas of the body at higher risk of infection with germ-fighting white blood cells.

**Try a supplement of vitamin E.** Research suggests that supplements of vitamin E may relieve symptoms, although how this works isn't completely understood. In various studies, people with intermittent claudication could walk farther and had better blood flow after taking 300 international units (I.U.) of vitamin E daily for three to six months. Many experts suggest taking 100 to 400 I.U. of vitamin E daily to help protect against various diseases, and this dose is considered safe.

**Take aspirin to help avoid arterial surgery.** Many doctors encourage people with claudication to use aspirin as part of a health-improvement program. A low-dose aspirin (325 milligrams) taken every other day may help you avoid the need for surgery, according to a study published in *Circulation*. Check with your physician, however, before taking regular doses of aspirin.

**Ask your doctor about surgery.** Among the surgical procedures typically used are balloon angioplasty, in which a catheter is inserted into the artery and a balloon is expanded within the artery to unblock the passageway, and atherectomy and arterial surgery, in which the plaque itself is removed or a length of the artery replaced with a clean vessel or tube.

### RAYNAUD'S DISEASE: FRIGID FINGERS AND TOES

Raynaud's phenomenon, or Raynaud's disease, occurs when blood flow to the fingers, toes and other parts of the body is dramatically reduced, causing abnormally cold fingers and toes. The condition afflicts nearly 10 percent of the population, but three-fourths of the sufferers are women, usually young or middle-aged.

If you've ever felt your fingers tingle and throb after taking a chair lift to the top of a ski trail while wearing gloves that weren't warm enough, you have some idea of what the condition feels like. But people with Raynaud's experience that kind of pain and numbness frequently. Most often, Raynaud's is brought on by cold temperatures or emotional stress, both of which can cause constricted blood vessels. It can last anywhere from a minute to several hours and affect one digit or all 20, according to Joseph M. Grisanti, M.D., assistant clinical professor of medicine at Millard Fillmore Hospital in Buffalo, New York. Raynaud's can also affect other parts of the body, such as the ears, nose, tongue and nipples.

The disease is associated with the use of certain drugs, including oral contraceptives, but it can also occur as a side effect of illnesses such as arthritis, arteriosclerosis or anemia. If you suffer from Raynaud's, some simple lifestyle changes may help control the condition.

**Stay away from stimulants.** Avoid caffeine, nicotine, decongestants and antihistamines—they constrict blood vessels and may increase both the frequency and the duration of episodes, says Dr. Grisanti.

**Avoid vibrations.** Raynaud's also turns up in 90 percent of workers in certain types of jobs—carpentry, construction and stone masonry, in particular. The common denominator is the use of tools that vibrate heavily, such as jackhammers, chainsaws and stone-cutting and -polishing machines, which can injure tiny blood vessels in the fingers and arms, reducing circulation throughout the hands. The cure might lie in giving the machine a rest. In extreme cases, a job change might be in order.

**Cover up.** Of course, the source of Raynaud's is not always so easily determined. Many who have the disease don't know what brought it on but are desperately looking for relief. Here are three common no-frills methods for dealing with Raynaud's.

- Wear gloves when reaching into the freezer or handling cold objects.
- Before going outside in cold weather, put on several layers of warm clothing.

• Use chemically or electrically warmed socks and gloves to warm extremities.

**Train your hands to triumph over temperature.** Other self-treatments for Raynaud's include training the vessels in the hands to say open even in chilly surroundings. Here are two methods described in the *Harvard Health Letter*.

While sitting or standing in a cold area, keep your hands in warm water. By doing this three to six times a day, every other day, for three or four weeks, you can teach the arteries in your fingers to remain open when your body is cold.

Or, through regular practice with biofeedback equipment, which can measure minute changes in body temperature, you can learn to alter the temperature in your fingers and other parts of your body. Studies show that this method is successful in reducing the onset of Raynaud's by 66 to 93 percent. The equipment is usually available to the general public through university programs and practicing clinical psychologists.

**Get in the swing of things.** Donald R. McIntyre, M.D., of Rutland, Vermont, has developed an effective anti-Raynaud's exercise that consists of swinging your arms in a circle. Begin as though throwing an underhand pitch, and simply follow through in a complete circle. The motion causes centrifugal force to send blood to the extremities and into constricted vessels of the hands and fingers, thus relieving the condition.

### PHLEBITIS: PAINFUL BUT PREVENTABLE

Phlebitis became a household word back when former President Richard Nixon developed the problem. This disease affects the venous system, the vessels that carry carbon-dioxide-laden blood back to the heart and lungs. These vessels can become inflamed or produce blood clots, making them swollen and tender and sometimes dangerous. Though most phlebitis sufferers experience only discomfort, even pain, in some cases a clot can travel to the lungs and cause a pulmonary embolism that could be fatal.

**ANTI-AGING CHECKUP**
# HOW'S YOUR CIRCULATION?

If you suspect you may have one of the circulatory problems described in this chapter, answer the following questions Yes or No.

\_\_\_\_ Do you experience frequent and persistent cramping in your calves and thighs after walking only a short distance, with pain so severe that you must sit until the discomfort disappears? This is a classic symptom of claudication, a consequence of poor circulation.

\_\_\_\_ Do you have abnormally cold toes and fingers consistently, with the coldness lasting from a few minutes to several hours (sometimes due to stress or cold temperatures)? This may be Raynaud's disease.

\_\_\_\_ Do you have discomfort or pain in one or both legs at rest? This may be venous disease, which can result from an injury to the leg, varicose veins, an infection or simple inactivity. A clot in the leg that can travel to the lungs and cause a pulmonary embolism is a danger here.

## INTERPRETING YOUR ANSWERS

Any of these symptoms call for a visit to your doctor. Circulatory problems respond well to therapy, which can enhance your quality of life and might save your life.

Phlebitis, also called thrombophlebitis, usually occurs in the legs. The most common causes are physical trauma (such as a blow to the leg), infection, inactivity or immobilization of an extremity, says Robert Ginsburg, M.D., a cardiologist and expert in vascular disorders at the University Hospital in Denver.

One of the best means of prevention is activity (with your doctor's okay). "If you stand or sit in the same position for long periods, you make it difficult for the veins, especially those in the legs to pump the blood back to the heart," says Dr. Ginsburg. "Veins are very sensitive to pressure. When the blood stagnates, it backs up into the valves within the vein and injures the vessel. Veins need muscles to help them pump the blood back to the heart, so the best thing you can do is periodically get up from your chair, walk around and do some leg lifts. That will get the blood pumping and take the pressure off the veins."

Talk to your doctor about drug therapy. He or she may want to prescribe heparin, an anticoagulant that dissolves clots.

*Editor's note:* You may have heard that aspirin assists blood flow through the arteries, but according to Dr. Ginsburg, there is no evidence as yet that it can be helpful in the treatment of phlebitis or venous problems. Ask your doctor before taking it.

# 10

# CONSTIPATION

Cure That Clogged-Up Feeling

**You** know you have problems when a bowel movement is something to celebrate.

Constipation is no laughing matter, however. It's extremely uncomfortable and can cause bloating, abdominal pain, fatigue, achiness and mental sluggishness as well. Stopped-up bowels can also lead to other problems, such as diverticulosis (sometimes painful pouches in the large intestine) or hemorrhoids. In addition, some scientists theorize that clogged-up intestines contribute to colon cancer and other woes because waste material languishes in the intestines so long.

## WHY WE GET CONSTIPATED

Irregularity is one modern ailment that we bring on entirely ourselves; it doesn't exist in less industrialized countries, points out Sherwood Gorbach, M.D., professor of medicine and community health at Tufts University School of Medicine in Boston. The problem started when people began to eat highly processed food and turn their noses up at fiber-rich beans and whole-grain breads. Fiber is an indigestible material that absorbs moisture, making feces softer and speeding them through the intestinal tract and out of the body. During the past 100 years, however, average fiber intake has fallen from about 40 grams a day to our current 15 to 20 grams a day. And, *not* coincidentally, constipation has become a common problem; in fact, Americans spend more than $400 million each year on laxatives.

Not that lack of fiber is the *only* culprit. Other things can contribute to constipation as well, including certain medications, travel, stress, premenstrual changes, pregnancy, hormonal imbalances and various diseases, lack of exercise and drinking too little water.

In most cases, constipation is relatively easy to vanquish by adopting simple lifestyle changes. (If the condition lingers for more than two to three weeks despite corrective action, consult your doctor.) Try these easy ways to bid adieu to constipation.

**Get on the fiber wagon.** Eating fiber doesn't just mean you have to sprinkle dry brown flakes on top of your food. Rodney Taylor, professor of medicine at the Royal Naval Hospital in Hampshire, England, suggests in the *British Medical Journal* that people increase their intake of vegetables, such as cabbage, carrots and apples. You should also eat more whole-wheat products, brown rice, root vegetables (potatoes, yams and parsnips), leafy greens and legumes such as beans, split peas and lentils—which is more like the diet our forebears ate before the industrial revolution.

Wheat bran is particularly effective at keeping your bowels moving well, though it may be a bit of a jolt for intestinal systems not accustomed to fibrous diets. In fact, you should proceed cautiously when introducing fiber into your diet. If you're not used to it, fiber can cause flatulence, distension and bloating. Make changes *gradually,* giving your intestinal bacteria time to adapt to the new regimen.

**Go when you need to go.** It may sound like simple advice, but in this hectic world, many of us tend to ignore the call of nature when we're busy. Try getting up a little earlier in the morning so that when the call comes, you have time to answer it.

**Unclog your bowels with exercise.** Regular bouts of exercise are a surefire way to get your bowels moving, as a South African study showed. Ten healthy adults between the ages of 22 and 41 were tested over three one-week periods, during which they either rested or bicycled or jogged an hour a day. During the resting phase, it took an average of 51.2 hours—

more than two days—for stools to move through the intestines. When the participants exercised daily, however, bowel transit time dropped to around 35 hours (about a day and a half).

Strength training can also help move things along. A study published in *Medicine and Science in Sports and Exercise* tested seven healthy, untrained men between the ages of 52 and 69. The men worked out on weight-lifting equipment three days a week for 13 weeks. On average, their stools sped through their bodies 56 percent faster than before they took up strength training.

**Drink heartily.** The drier your stool, the harder it is to eliminate. "People need adequate water to maintain healthy elimination," says Marvin Schuster, M.D., chief of the division of digestive diseases and professor of medicine at Johns Hopkins University School of Medicine in Baltimore. This is especially important for older people or anyone who works hard physically or exercises often. Four to six glasses of water a day is usually adequate, says Dr. Schuster, but more is fine. (You can't count coffee, cola or tea: These beverages are diuretics, which actually cause you to lose water.)

**Check out those pills you're popping.** Many over-the-counter supplements or medications can cause constipation. These include iron and calcium supplements, antacids that contain calcium and medications or antacids that contain aluminum, including AlternaGel, Amphojel, Benadryl, Gaviscon, Maalox, Mylanta, Rolaids and many nighttime pain formulations.

**For some action, try prunes.** "Prunes do work as laxatives," says Dr. Schuster. Prunes irritate the bowel, stimulating peristalsis, the rhythmic contraction and expansion of the muscles of the walls of the large intestine that moves feces through the bowel and out. The fruit also contains fiber, which enhances the laxative effects. But prunes should be reserved for occasional jump starts, caution experts, so your bowels don't become dependent on them.

**Use laxatives as a last resort.** Doctors warn against turning to laxatives. "Used regularly, all methods of purging the bowel, enemas as well as laxatives, tend to weaken bowel function and cause dependence," states Marvin M. Lipman,

M.D., in *Consumer Reports Health Letter*. "Laxatives should be avoided if possible, or used only occasionally."

If you do feel the need for a laxative, avoid chemical varieties. Instead, reach for a bulk-forming laxative, such as one made with psyllium. This high-fiber seed draws water into the stool, which makes it larger, softer and much easier to move along.

---

**ANTI-AGING CHECKUP**
# HOW HEALTHY ARE YOUR BOWEL HABITS?

Wondering if you're constipated or if you have a problem that warrants seeing a doctor? Check off the statements that apply to you, then study the interpretations below.

_____ 1. You never move your bowels two days in a row.
_____ 2. You have fewer than three bowel movements a week and have difficulty passing stools.
_____ 3. Your stools are always small and hard.
_____ 4. You always have to strain to have a bowel movement.
_____ 5. You see blood or red matter in your stools.
_____ 6. Blood sometimes drips from your rectum.

**INTERPRETING YOUR ANSWERS**

1. This doesn't mean you're constipated; everyone's schedule is different. "There is no magic number of bowel movements per day, or per week, that would indicate what is 'normal' or whether you are constipated," says Marvin Schuster, M.D., chief of the division of digestive diseases and professor of medicine at Johns Hopkins University School of Medicine in Baltimore. "Some people go once a day; some, once every three days."
2. You're probably constipated. Increase your fiber intake, drink more water and get some exercise.

*continued*

3. This is a definite indication that you're constipated. Again, increase your fiber and water intake and exercise more often.
4. Sounds like you're constipated. The solution is probably as simple as upping your intake of fiber and water and scheduling a daily hike around the neighborhood.
5. This could be the harmless result of eating red-colored food (such as beets), or it could indicate a serious condition warranting immediate attention. See your doctor.
6. This could be due to a slight tear in the skin around your anus, or it could be from hemorrhoids, intestinal infections, ulcerative colitis, Crohn's disease, diverticula or changes in blood vessels due to aging. It can suggest the presence of benign colorectal polyps and cancer in the colon. See your doctor.

# 11

# DIABETES

Top Strategies for Fighting Back

**Diabetes** is nothing to ignore. It doubles the risk of heart disease and the chances of suffering a stroke. In addition, diabetes dramatically increases the rates of kidney disease, blindness from retinopathy, and infection and complications during childbearing.

But this grim picture can be often avoided. Diabetes in adults can be prevented in most cases, and many of those who already have the disease can live healthy lives, according to physicians. Others can substantially reduce the risk of suffering the side effects of diabetes. All of this can be accomplished by lifestyle changes alone—changes that will not only improve the quality of life but may extend it, too.

## UNSCRAMBLING DIABETES: TYPES I AND II

Diabetes prevents the body from utilizing glucose or blood sugar, which is derived from food and carried to cells by insulin, a hormone produced by the pancreas. Insulin permits glucose to enter the cell, where it is used as fuel.

Of the nation's 13 million people with diabetes, approximately 90 percent suffer from Type II, non-insulin-dependent diabetes mellitus. This disease, usually contracted in adulthood and called adult-onset diabetes, seldom requires daily insulin injections. Instead, it may often be controlled with diet alone or with oral drugs that enhance insulin function.

In the early stages of Type II diabetes, the body produces

more insulin than normal, but that can dwindle to a dangerous low over time. "Type II diabetics go through a natural history," says Stephen Inkeles, M.D., an internist at the Pritikin Longevity Center in Santa Monica, California. "As the disease progresses, the pancreas secretes less and less insulin. Eventually, they may need insulin injections."

The remaining 10 percent of people with diabetes have Type I, juvenile diabetes, which usually appears in childhood. People with Type I diabetes do not produce any insulin and require regular injections.

The Pritikin Longevity Center has demonstrated the value of diet and exercise in overcoming diabetes for thousands of sufferers. Ninety percent of people with diabetes on oral medication leave the center no longer needing those drugs. Of those who arrive taking insulin, 50 percent leave insulin-free.

You don't have to go to a center, hospital or spa to achieve these results. Working with your doctor, you can improve your health right in your own home.

### REACH FOR THE COMPLEX CARBOHYDRATES

Make sure that 50 to 60 percent of your total calories come from foods rich in complex carbohydrates, such as whole grains, bread, pasta, potatoes, vegetables and fruit, says the American Diabetes Association. Failing to meet this goal can be hazardous. A study published in the *American Journal of Epidemiology* showed that a person with diabetes who drops just 90 grams of complex carbs daily from his or her diet can increase the risk of impaired glucose tolerance by 56 percent. (Ninety grams would be the equivalent of one sweet potato, a cup of macaroni and cheese and a slice of French bread.)

"Complex carbohydrates are broken down slowly in the intestines and take longer to get into the bloodstream," says Dr. Inkeles. They provide a consistent flow of energy, without the extreme peaks and valleys in blood sugar that occur when you eat refined white sugar. Try these strategies to ensure you get enough of complex carbs every day.

**Increase your fiber intake.** A fringe benefit of eating complex carbohydrates is the added fiber you get, which makes a big difference in how your body handles sugar. "Fiber slows absorption of carbohydrates even further by slowing digestion," says Dr. Inkeles. "Consequently, the glucose is absorbed gradually." The fiber in fresh fruit works the same way—it slows absorption of sugars and thus balances blood sugar levels.

**Chow down on oatmeal.** "The ideal breakfast for a person with diabetes is hot oatmeal," says Dr. Inkeles, "because it combines the complex carbohydrates with the soluble fiber." A whole-grain breakfast also provides enduring energy throughout the morning.

**Grazing is good for you.** Research shows that blood sugar levels remain consistently balanced when people eat three square meals plus two or three healthful snacks per day. "Ideally, a person with diabetes can eat up to six meals a day: three standard meals and two or three small ones," says Dr. Inkeles. In his opinion, the best snacks are vegetables, whole grains and breads, beans and peas and occasionally fruit. The best fruit? "Apples, pears and berries, because of their fiber content, which will also help stabilize glucose levels," he says.

## TRIM THE FAT FROM YOUR DIET

The typical American diet is rich in fat, which raises the risk of getting diabetes. Research shows that for every extra 40 grams of fat you eat per day—the amount in a 4-ounce hamburger with a large order of fries—you triple your risk of contracting Type II diabetes.

Four times as many second-generation Japanese-American men have Type II diabetes as Japanese men living in Japan, according to a study published by the American Society of Clinical Nutrition. Researchers examined the diets and health patterns of 229 Japanese-American men, whose diets were a little too American for their own good. The residents of Japan, however, ate a standard diet of miso soup, rice, fish and vegetables. While both groups ate about the same number of calories, the Japanese-Americans got far more of their calories from fat. The result: an epidemic of diabetes among the Americans.

How can you lower the amount of fat in your diet? Steer clear of fried foods and high-fat dairy products. Choose low-fat or nonfat milk and cheeses; skip the sour cream, butter and ice cream. Remove the skin from poultry, and trim all visible fat from meat. Study labels, and choose low-fat products over high-fat ones (pretzels, for example, instead of potato chips).

Cutting dietary fat, combined with an exercise program, will also help you lose weight. And not only will that improve all aspects of health for the overweight diabetic, it may be enough by itself to overcome the need for medication and insulin, according to research published in *Choices in Cardiology*. People with diabetes, especially those with Type II, commonly suffer from obesity. But studies show that losing weight lowers blood glucose levels, blood lipids, blood pressure and protein losses from the kidneys. Normalization of weight also improves muscle and joint function and reduces the risk of surgery.

## Discover the Magic Nutrients Can Do

People with diabetes have been found deficient in a variety of nutrients, particularly the B vitamins riboflavin, vitamin $B_6$ and folate. Now scientists believe that a lack of certain nutrients may play a pivotal role in the onset and development of the disease.

**Consider chromium.** Adequate levels of chromium may prevent mild glucose intolerance from becoming Type II diabetes. Researchers examined the effects of supplementary chromium on 17 people, 8 with mild glucose intolerance, a condition that may escalate to diabetes. Half of the 17 took 200 micrograms of chromium daily for five weeks; the others took placebos with no chromium. Then the two groups switched pills so that those who had received the placebos now got the chromium. When the glucose-intolerant people were given a sugar drink, their sugar levels rose only half as high during the period that they were taking chromium as when they weren't.

Americans typically consume an average of 30 micrograms of chromium per day. This does not mean that you have to start taking supplements to increase your intake. Rather, doctors recommend that you cut down on foods such as simple sugars, found in pastries, sodas and other sweets, which deplete the chromium content of your blood. Instead, eat more chromium "preservers," particularly complex carbohydrates in whole grains, vegetables, pastas and potatoes.

**Magnesium may help.** When elderly people with insulin resistance were given 4.5 grams of magnesium daily for four weeks, their glucose metabolism improved significantly, reported the *American Journal of Clinical Nutrition*. The researchers think that extra magnesium helps regulate age-related changes in both blood chemistry and glucose handling. You can also get magnesium naturally in foods such as nuts, legumes, whole grains, bananas and green vegetables.

**Ask your doctor about niacin.** When a derivative of the B vitamin niacin, called nicotinamide, was given to 14 children on the verge of developing diabetes, only 1 child contracted the disease. Eight other predisposed children who did not receive the drug developed diabetes, reported *Diabetologia*.

"The results are dramatic," says Peter Chase, M.D., of the Barbara Davis Center for Childhood Diabetes at the University of Colorado Health Sciences Center in Denver. "But the study needs to be repeated with more subjects to see if the results are really valid." Researchers believe that nicotinamide interferes with the destruction of certain cells in the pancreas that cause diabetes in children.

*Warning:* Niacin itself may actually be dangerous to people with Type II diabetes, especially if consumed in the high quantities typical of those who take the nutrient to lower cholesterol. When researchers gave niacin to people with Type II diabetes, it raised blood sugar levels by 16 percent. Blood levels of uric acid also rose, suggesting probable kidney problems and increased risk of gout. There's no danger from niacin in your diet, however—you can't get enough of it from food to cause a reaction.

### GET THE GLUCOSE TRANSPORTERS GOING

Aerobic exercise—such as walking, jogging, swimming, tennis or cycling—may prevent people with impaired glucose tolerance from becoming diabetic.

Insulin, which is supposed to deliver glucose to cells, is often blocked in people with diabetes. Consequently, the glucose doesn't get to the cells in the quantities required for normal functioning. This causes blood sugar levels to rise dangerously, resulting in all the aforementioned side effects.

Exercise removes the roadblocks that prevent insulin from delivering glucose to cells. Aerobic exercise boosts the production of the proteins that pull glucose into the muscles, according to research led by William J. Evans, Ph.D., director of Noll Laboratory for Human Performance and professor of nutrition at Pennsylvania State University in University Park and coauthor of inside *Biomarkers: The 10 Determinants of Aging You Can Control*. Once inside the muscles, the glucose can be burned as energy or stored as fuel. Tufts scientists have shown that aerobic training actually increases the level of one of those protein transporters, called GLUT 4. By enabling the body to handle sugar more efficiently, exercise also helps regulate insulin production and keeps energy levels more balanced. Three or four exercise sessions a week are best.

Regular exercise speeds metabolism, says Dr. Inkeles, which causes blood sugar to be burned more efficiently, even while you are resting.

**Go the extra mile.** According to Susan P. Helmrich, Ph.D., an epidemiologist at the University of California, Berkeley, "putting a little extra oomph in your daily walk could have a real impact against developing the disease."

Dr. Helmrich studied the effects of exercise on 5,990 men over 14 years. "We found that men who exercised regularly prevented or delayed the onset of the disease," she says. For every 500 calories burned during a week, your risk of developing Type II diabetes may drop 6 percent. (It takes about 60 minutes of vigorous exercise to burn 500 calories.)

People with diabetes tend to have high triglycerides, which are harmful blood fats, and low levels of the "good" cholesterol, HDL—and hence have an increased risk of heart disease. As exercise burns triglycerides in the blood and raises HDL, there are multiple benefits to exercise.

**Pump a little iron.** Resistance training, such as weight lifting, also speeds metabolism, which will cause your body to burn calories even while you're relaxing. Also, muscle is a big calorie-consumer, while fat just serves as a storehouse for calories. The more muscle you have, the more your body burns the glucose in your blood.

Resistance training also improves your body's sensitivity to insulin, so less insulin is needed to handle the sugar in the blood. In one study involving 15 men—6 young, 9 elderly— *all* of the participants showed improved insulin efficiency after 12 weeks of weight training. Therefore, the men did not have to produce higher quantities of insulin to metabolize the glucose in their blood. (For more on weight training, see chapters 13 and 32.)

Like aerobics, resistance training lowers LDL cholesterol (the type that causes atherosclerosis, increasing the risk of heart disease) and elevates the helpful HDL.

Researchers from Johns Hopkins University and the University of Maryland recruited 37 men and divided them into three groups: One group jogged, another took up strength training, and a third didn't exercise. After 18 weeks, each group was given glucose tolerance tests, which reveal how efficiently the body uses blood sugar. Both the joggers and the weight lifters saw significant improvement, while the nonexercisers experienced no improvement. Remarkably, 3 of the 4 prediabetic people who participated in strength training saw their glucose tolerance return to normal.

*Editor's note:* People with diabetes should check with their doctor before beginning an exercise program because their risk of heart disease is much higher than average.

## ANTI-AGING CHECKUP
# THE OFFICIAL DIABETES QUIZ

The American Diabetes Association (ADA) provides the following self-test for people to grade their own risk of contracting diabetes. Answer each of the following questions Yes or No.

1. I have been experiencing mone or more of the following symptoms on a regular basis.
   ____ a. Excessive thirst
   ____ b. Frequent urination
   ____ c. Extreme fatigue
   ____ d. Unexplained weight loss
   ____ e. Blurry vision periodically
____ 2. I am over 30 years old.
____ 3. My weight is 20 percent over the maximum ideal weight for my height.
____ 4. I am a woman who has had more than one baby weighing more than 9 pounds at birth.
____ 5. I am of Native American descent.
____ 6. I am of Latino or African-American descent.
____ 7. I have one or both parent(s) with diabetes.
____ 8. I have a brother or sister with diabetes.

## INTERPRETING YOUR ANSWERS

For every Yes answer, give yourself the following number of points. For No answers, you receive no points.

| | | |
|---|---|---|
| 1a.  3 points | 1e.  2 points | 5.  1 point |
| 1b.  3 points | 2.  1 point | 6.  1 point |
| 1c.  1 point | 3.  2 points | 7.  1 point |
| 1d.  3 points | 4.  2 points | 8.  2 points |

**Total:** _____

If you score between 3 and 5 points, you are probably at low risk of getting diabetes. However, if your score is above 5, you may be at high risk or may already have diabetes. The best thing to do is see your doctor soon.

The ADA is quick to point out that if you have any suspicion of illness, you should see your doctor, no matter what your score.

# 12

# DIVERTICULAR DISEASE

A Simple Solution
for a 20th-Century Ailment

**Chances** are your great-grandparents didn't have this sometimes painful and potentially serious gastrointestinal ailment. But today 65 percent of Americans 85 and older have diverticulosis, the mild form of diverticular disease, says Atilla Ertan, M.D., chief of gastroenterology at Baylor College of Medicine in Houston.

Why? The answer revolves around diet. Chances are your great-grandparents ate plenty of whole grains, beans and vegetables. In contrast, today many of us eat fewer fibrous foods and more processed white flour and meat, which tend to clog things up in the intestines. We have smaller, harder stools, and our intestines have to squeeze mightily to keep things moving along. Eventually, something gives.

It's sort of like squeezing a balloon, says Sherwood Gorbach, M.D., professor of medicine and community health at Tufts University School of Medicine in Boston. "You get a lot of pressure in the place you squeeze, but a swollen or balloon effect in the other places."

The result is that diverticula—small, usually pea-size bulges or pockets—form in the large intestine. This is called diverticulosis. These bulges generally appear in the sigmoid colon, the lowest part of the colon, near the rectum. The sufferer might have painful attacks in the lower-left part of the body follow-

ng a meal or when passing gas. Sometimes a blood vessel in
ne of the bulges will tear, causing rectal bleeding that requires medical treatment.

More seriously, the diverticula can become infected and
esult in a condition known as diverticulosis, causing fever,
abdominal cramps, tenderness, diarrhea or constipation. While
antibiotics can cure the problem, if untreated it can progress to
peritonitis, a life-threatening condition.

## Sidestep Diverticular Problems

The good news is that this potentially painful disorder is
completely avoidable. Yes, as you get older, the walls of your
intestine grow a bit weaker, which is why diverticular disease
seldom occurs in people under 40. Fiber, however, can prevent
he problem: It absorbs water and swells in the intestine, form-
ng large, soft feces that require a minimum of pressure to
move them along the colon, so there is less chance of a
"blowout."

Only surgery can eliminate diverticula that already exist,
but you can prevent new ones from forming. The following
program will help ensure a healthy intestine, says Dr. Ertan.

**Munch more fiber.** Dr. Ertan says people with diverticular
disease should consume 25 to 30 grams of fiber per day, an
amount a varied diet easily provides. Among the best sources
of fiber are whole grains, such as brown rice, wheat and corn,
vegetables, fruits and nuts, plus bran sprinkled on foods. An
orange has about 3 grams of fiber, a bowl of bran cereal has
about 6 grams, and a serving of kidney beans contains about 7
grams. (You should ease back on your fiber intake during a
flare-up of the disease, however.)

**Drink water, water and more water.** Dr. Ertan recommends eight to ten glasses of water per day to help keep the
stool soft. "Unfortunately, Americans have a bad habit of
neglecting water," he says. "It's especially important in the
summertime or for people living in hot southern climates."

**Move your body.** Walk daily for 30 to 45 minutes, recommends Dr. Ertan. The exercise helps stimulate your bowels,
and walking lets gravity do its part, too. If walking bores you,

try bicycling or any other aerobic activity to get things moving.

**Forget about laxatives.** While constipation can raise pressure in the colon, increasing the risk of diverticulosis, the regular use of chemical laxatives may also weaken the intestines and contribute to diverticular problems, according to the National Digestive Diseases Information Clearinghouse. Instead, depend on a fiber-rich diet with plenty of water and exercise to avoid constipation.

**Take your time in the john.** "Research shows that Americans are in too big a hurry when they sit on the toilet. It's better to take a newspaper or magazine into the bathroom, relax, and spend 10 to 15 minutes more to help the large bowel fully empty," said Dr. Ertan. Don't strain—just relax and let nature take its course.

**ANTI-AGING CHECKUP**
# PAINS YOU SHOULDN'T IGNORE

If you have small bulges in your intestines, a condition known as diverticulosis, symptoms may not occur unless the bulges become infected (called diverticulitis). To check out the state of your intestines, answer these questions Yes or No.

_____ Do you have pain in the lower-left quadrant of the body, perhaps with cramps that radiate to the back?

_____ Do you feel tenderness and muscle spasms in the stomach wall, especially on the left side?

_____ Are you frequently constipated?

_____ Do your stools contain mucus or blood?

_____ Do you have fever, accompanied by chills and nausea?

_____ Do you frequently feel the urgent need to urinate? (About 10 percent of people with diverticulitis experience this, caused by the swollen colon pressing against the bladder.)

**INTERPRETING YOUR ANSWERS**

If you answered more than one of these questions Yes, check with your doctor; diverticulitis requires treatment with antibiotics. If you have no signs of intestinal problems, however, follow the steps recommended in this chapter to *keep* your intestines healthy.

# 13

# ENDURANCE

### Building Stamina Step-by-Step

**The** myths surrounding the human body seem endless, but few hang on so stubbornly as the notion that we automatically lose our endurance as we get older. Don't believe it. Studies show that men and women of all ages—even those well into their 80s—can improve endurance substantially and forestall the aging process. The secret: just a little regular exercise, three or four times per week.

"Endurance is the amount of time you can sustain a given power output," says Michael Stone, Ph. D., an exercise physiologist at Appalachian State University in Boone, North Carolina. For most of us, that means our ability to walk, run, lift objects or work without feeling weak or tired.

### BUILDING BLOOD VESSELS

It's true that as we get older, we tend to tire more quickly. But that kind of fatigue is not necessarily related to age.

As muscles work harder, they need more oxygen and nutrients to perform their tasks. They also produce more waste products, such as carbon dioxide and lactic acid, which accumulate within the muscle tissue if they're not eliminated.

Oxygen and nutrients are delivered and waste removed through the body's vast network of blood vessels, especially its tiniest vessels called capillaries. Capillaries serve as the body's indoor plumbing, delivering the stuff your cells require

nd removing what they need to get rid of. Consequently, the
nore capillaries you have, the greater your endurance!

These capillaries tend to shrink or even disappear if you be-
ome sedentary. Luckily, the process can be reserved with ex-
rcise. The more active you are, the more capillaries you grow
o deliver more oxygen and nutrients and eliminate more
vaste—thus eliminating the underlying causes of fatigue.

Exercise also prompts your heart to pump more blood per
eat and your lungs to enrich your blood with greater quanti-
ies of oxygen. The net effect: You look and feel younger and
tronger.

## MATCH YOUR EXERCISE TO YOUR GOALS

To build endurance, exercise physiologists recommend a
vide variety of exercises and activities, from gardening to aer-
bic training (such as walking, jogging and bicycling) to
naerobic exercises (such as weight training).

"The kind of program you choose depends upon what you
vant to strengthen and the kinds of work you do," says Dr.
tone. "If you do a job that requires you to lift heavy objects,
ou want to improve your muscle endurance and your ability
o lift. For that, a weight program is best. But if you sit behind
 desk and want to improve your cardiovascular and pul-
nonary systems, then you probably want to do some aerobic
raining."

Bryant Stamford, Ph.D., an exercise physiologist and direc-
or of the Health Promotion and Wellness Center in Louisville,
Kentucky, agrees: "You develop endurance for specific tasks,
nd there isn't much crossover. Swimming does not improve a
unner's endurance for running. The key is to do the things
ou like doing regularly or are being asked to do."

Dr. Stamford, who is the author of *Fitness without Exercise*,
ays that all the activities a person needs to improve endurance
lready exist in the course of a normal week. "If someone
ikes to garden, I say, 'Fine. Garden an hour a day, three times
 week. Now what else? Are there some stairs in your apart-
nent or house? Walk up and down those stairs a few times a
lay.' That same person may say he likes to walk in the park or
ick a soccer ball or walk to work. The activities that are fun

and easy are the ideal ways of developing fitness and endurance."

## COMBINE ANAEROBIC WITH AEROBIC

For those seeking a specific program, the American College of Sports Medicine recommends a combination of aerobic training—exercises that increase the flow of oxygen to your muscles—and anaerobic training—exercises that utilize the oxygen already present in your muscle tissue. Anaerobic exercise is generally referred to as resistance training, meaning the use of free weights, machine or the weight of your body.

**Add wrist weights.** There are lots of ways to combine aerobic and anaerobic activities. For example, many people take a brisk walk while wearing wrist weights. Studies show that combining brisk walking with a pound or two of wrist weights can lower blood pressure in people with hypertension, even elderly men and women. (If you're being treated for high blood pressure, check with your doctor before exercising with weights of any kind.)

**Join a club.** Health clubs or your local Y offer not only exercise equipment such as treadmills, stationary bicycles, stair climbers, rowers and cross-country ski machines—any of which would help improve your endurance—but also have all kinds of weight machines for strength training.

## WARM UP, COOL DOWN AND LISTEN TO YOUR BODY

Before beginning any vigorous exercise program, you'll want to consult a physician if you have one or more risk factors for heart disease, such as smoking, elevated blood cholesterol, high blood pressure or a history of heart disease.

And before starting to exercise, you should do some warm-ups, especially if you are over 50. It's important not to stretch cold muscles, so experts recommend that you start out by walking at a slow to moderate pace for five to ten minutes, then pause to do some stretching exercises. After that, walk at a brisk pace or proceed with your exercise program, then cool down with more slow walking and light stretching.

Ideally, you eventually want to burn about 285 calories per

exercise session, which is the equivalent of walking three miles. But you can improve endurance with much less, especially if you're unfit.

As you exercise, listen to your body. If you're panting vigorously, slow down. If you can't hold a conversation, take a break. If your muscles are in agony, back off. It's better to work not quite hard enough than to push too hard.

---

**ANTI-AGING CHECKUP**
## KEEPING TRACK OF YOUR HEART RATE

Once your physician has given you the go-ahead for an exercise program, monitor your heart rate to ensure that you get the most benefit from each session. Ideally, you want to your heart rate to reach between 60 and 85 percent of its maximum, according to the American College of Sports Medicine.

To determine your maximum heart rate, subtract your age from 220. If you are 50 years old, your maximum heart rate would be 170. For the most benefit from an exercise session, a 50-year-old should get his or her heart rate up between 112 and 145 beats per minute and keep it there for 15 to 20 minutes.

Measure your heart rate by putting your fingers on the radial artery at the wrist. Many athletes check their pulse by pressing on the carotid artery at the neck, but massaging it too vigorously can instantly slow down your heart rate and cause you to underestimate the exertion of your workout.

# 14

# ENERGY

## How to Sharpen Your Edge

**Are** you suffering from your own personal energy crisis?

Many of us get out of bed feeling like we're still under a blanket of fatigue and don't hit our mid-morning energy peak until we've been jump-started by a couple of cups of coffee. The rest of the day is a pattern of energy swells and dips. We coast through late morning and early afternoon, find ourselves flagging after lunch, rally for another hour or two, and then turn into mush at about 3:00 P.M. That's the "heartbreak hill" of the day, the point at which we have to fight to keep our eyes open or rely on repeated jolts of java, with its inevitable side effects of jitters, irritability and midnight wakefulness.

High energy, all day and every day, is the Holy Grail of good health. We experience energy as physical vitality, mental alertness and creativity. Yet, at its most elemental level, energy is life. Reduce our energy, and we are less than the sum of our parts. Too few of us realize what a rich supply of energy we do possess, and even fewer know that we can all raise these energy levels still higher without turning to the coffeepot.

"No one fully understands why we get tired," says Robert Thayer, Ph.D., a psychologist at California State University, Long Beach, and an expert of human energy. "There seem to be biological rhythms that we are all subject to. These are repetitive energy patterns that differ among individuals, but we all seem to have good hours and poor hours. What our research has shown is that you can improve your energy levels, even during your poor hours." Dr. Thayer and other energy experts point out that there are at least five areas of life—sleep, exercise, enthusiasm, diet and body rhythms—that directly affect our energy levels, and we can influence all of them.

## THE GIFTS OF A GOOD NIGHT'S SLEEP

Sleep is the first thing most of us cut back on when we're pressed for time, but that loss can dramatically affect how we feel and perform. "We are sleeping an hour a day less than we were in 1900," says Richard Podell, M.D., of the Robert Wood Johnson Medical School in New Brunswick, New Jersey. An hour of lost sleep will reduce alertness by as much as 20 percent the next day. Even worse, the losses add up, so that after sleep-deprived nights, your alertness can be diminished by as much as 50 percent, says Timothy Roehrs, Ph.D., director of research at Henry Ford Hospital's Sleep Disorders and Research Center in Detroit.

Hours in bed do not of themselves define quality sleep, however. "Sleep is often disturbed by waking up in the middle of the night or remaining awake for half an hour or more," says Dr. Podell. To avoid disruptions, he urges people to abstain from caffeine and alcohol in the evenings and before bed. Both substances make it difficult for the body to relax and enter deep sleep.

Just as lost sleep diminishes our energy, additional sleep can heighten it. Adding an extra hour of sleep, for example, can increase your daytime alertness by a third, says Dr. Roehrs. That's the energy equivalent of two cups of coffee.

Such a benefit can be derived only by going to bed an hour earlier, however. Sleeping late, perhaps on Saturday or Sunday morning, throws off your biological clock and can actually increase drowsiness, especially when reality—7:00 A.M.—hits on Monday morning.

## THE EXERCISE SECRET

You may think that exercise will tire you out, but aerobic activities actually *give* you energy. They can also bestow an array of other treasures upon you. "Moderate exercise has a body-wide effect, arousing a number of different systems," says Dr. Thayer. "The primary effect is energy enhancement, the secondary effect is tension reduction, and the third effect is increased optimism and an improvement of mood about the future." Try the following to give yourself a boost.

**Take a walk.** A ten-minute walk at any time of the day will work wonders. "Our research has shown that a ten-minute walk—even during the mid- to late-afternoon hours, when your energy has fallen—can raise your energy levels to those of your high-energy periods, such as mid-morning," says Dr. Thayer. And that burst of new energy can last for one to two hours.

**Do it regularly.** All aerobic exercises—walking, running and dancing—will increase the amount of oxygen in your bloodstream and muscles. Work our 20 to 40 minutes a day, three to five days a week, to increase your energy levels.

**Squeeze in activity.** Exercise physiologists recommend that we fit some aerobic exercise into our daily routine. If possible, walk to work or to meetings outside your office building. Garden, take the stairs instead of the elevator, or enjoy a brisk walk during your lunch hour. Short bursts of exercise will release untapped energy reserves.

### Enthusiasm Equals Energy

"We know that mood and attitude are related to the secretion of certain chemicals in the brain," says Joseph Hellige, Ph.D., professor of psychology at the University of Southern California in Los Angeles. "And these changes in brain chemistry can influence how much energy we experience."

Within certain limits, even stress can boost your energy, especially if you regard your task as a challenge and an opportunity. But prolonged anxiety, tension and stress can drain energy and, even worse, lead to depression. "There's no question that people who are depressed experience much-lower-than-normal levels of energy," says Jaak Panksepp, Ph.D., professor of psychobiology at Bowling Green State University in Ohio. On the other hand, excitement and optimism are known to increase energy levels. Here's how to add some spice to your life.

**Keep friendships alive.** When you're drained of energy or overloaded with work, you may be tempted to keep to yourself. Wrong move, say the experts. Friendships or a good relationship with your spouse can help you over the hurdles. People who have close and supportive relationships experience greater energy.

**Give of yourself.** Something that researchers call helper's high—greater energy and enhanced self-esteem—appears to result from acts of altruism. Scientists speculate that aiding others may cause the brain to secrete endorphins, opium-like substances that stimulate feelings of well-being, heighten awareness, energy and joy.

**Find the silver lining.** Simply think positively, and your body will experience a reduction of tension, which can improve circulation and enhance energy levels.

**Channel your energy.** Finally, the energy experts recommend that you avoid thinking of energy as a limited resource to be guarded or preserved. Instead, give yourself freely to the task at hand, and you'll find yourself experiencing greater vitality. "If you're alive, you've got energy. Use it, conserve it and channel it in the right way, and you'll seem to have more," says Kenneth Bruscia, Ph.D., professor at Temple University in Philadelphia.

### FOOD FOR THOUGHT

If you're starting your day with jelly doughnuts and half a pot of coffee, well, no wonder you find yourself lagging later. We all know that food is fuel, but some foods make better fuel than others.

**Choose complex carbs.** Your best bets in the carbohydrate department are whole grains, such as brown rice, barley, millet and corn, whole-wheat bread, pasta and potatoes.

**Load up on nutrients.** No, not the stuff in bottles—the vitamins and minerals you find in foods. You get vitamin C in citrus fruits and leafy greens, B vitamins in brown rice and leafy greens, and potassium and magnesium in beans, potatoes, leafy greens and fruit.

**Get your iron.** You'll find this essential mineral in figs, prunes, raisins, beans, leafy greens, fish and meat. Since iron is essential for the transport of oxygen by red blood cells, deficiencies can cause fatigue.

**Steer clear of dietary fat.** Foods high in fat, such as french fries, butter, fatty cuts of meat and rich pastries or desserts, can actually rob us of energy. The same is true of excesses of coffee and alcohol.

**Watch your sugar intake.** Limit soft drinks and foods rich in sugar. "Most people think that sugar causes an increase in energy, and, in fact, it does work temporarily, but sugar has an insidious effect. It depletes energy after an hour or so," says Dr. Thayer. "We compared the energy increase resulting from a ten-minute walk versus a candy bar and found that after an hour, the people who ate the candy bar has less energy than those who took the walk. Not only that, but the people who ate the candy bar had increased levels of tension."

**Eat protein for an energy boost.** Dr. Podell recommends that people eat a light lunch that includes a low-fat protein source such as turkey, tuna or low-fat yogurt. The lunchtime protein may enhance both energy and brain activity during the afternoon.

### FINDING YOUR RHYTHM

We each have our own daily energy patterns, which scientists refer to as circadian rhythms. Dr. Thayer recommends that we become aware of our energy peaks and valleys and, whenever possible, schedule the most stressful challenges during high-energy periods.

While there are individual differences, people typically peak at mid-morning, between 10:00 A.M. and noon. There's often a dip after lunch, especially if you've eaten a heavy meal. This is followed by a rise in energy around 2:00 P.M. and a steep fall at 3:00 or 4:00 P.M. A subpeak emerges at about 6:00 or 7:00 P.M., after which you steadily lose energy, mental sharpness and alertness.

Ideally, most of us would take a brief nap in early afternoon. If you work a regular schedule, however, you likely can't. So what can you do if your natural fatigue falls during a period when you have to be alert and busy? Try a brisk walk, improve what you eat, and schedule your least demanding tasks during your less alert periods. It may also help to switch to a different task.

If your fatigue continues to linger, however, it could indicate any of a number of serious illnesses and should be checked out by a physician. Otherwise, a lack of energy is a manageable, all-too-human phenomenon.

---

**ANTI-AGING CHECKUP**
# FOLLOW YOUR BODY RHYTHMS

Keep a journal to note your energy fluctuations. Rate your energy levels on a scale of 1 to 10 (1 being an almost total lack of energy, 10 being the peak) every hour or so. Track these peaks and valleys for a few days. Then tackle your more demanding tasks when your know you're about to enter an energy surge.

| TIME OF DAY | ENERGY LEVEL (ON A SCALE OF 1 TO 10) | | |
| --- | --- | --- | --- |
| | DAY 1 | DAY 2 | DAY 3 |
| 6:00 A.M. | _____ | _____ | _____ |
| 7:00 A.M. | _____ | _____ | _____ |
| 8:00 A.M. | _____ | _____ | _____ |
| 9:00 A.M. | _____ | _____ | _____ |
| 10:00 A.M. | _____ | _____ | _____ |
| 11:00 A.M. | _____ | _____ | _____ |
| 12:00 NOON | _____ | _____ | _____ |
| 1:00 P.M. | _____ | _____ | _____ |
| 2:00 P.M. | _____ | _____ | _____ |
| 3:00 P.M. | _____ | _____ | _____ |
| 4:00 P.M. | _____ | _____ | _____ |
| 5:00 P.M. | _____ | _____ | _____ |
| 6:00 P.M. | _____ | _____ | _____ |
| 7:00 P.M. | _____ | _____ | _____ |
| 8:00 P.M. | _____ | _____ | _____ |
| 9:00 P.M. | _____ | _____ | _____ |
| 10:00 P.M. | _____ | _____ | _____ |
| 11:00 P.M. | _____ | _____ | _____ |
| 12:00 MIDNIGHT | _____ | _____ | _____ |
| 1:00 A.M. | _____ | _____ | _____ |

# 15

# FLEXIBILITY

### Use It or Lose It

**Remember** when you thought nothing about touching your toes without bending your knees? Today you may find it tough, if not impossible, to get those fingers down to the toes without pain.

You may think of this loss of suppleness as inevitable. But it's not—and retaining our flexibility is more crucial to our health, mobility and future than many of us realize.

"As we lose flexibility, we lose range of motion, and normal movements become more restricted and painful," says William Cornelius, Ph.D., associate professor of physical education at the University of North Texas. "As people lose normal range of motion, they become less mobile. Also, loss of flexibility is associated with greater incidence of injuries."

The good news is that much of our flexibility can be retained and lost flexibility regained. In fact, regaining lost flexibility is one of the keys to staying young.

### FLEXIBILITY KEEPS YOU YOUNG

First, since most of us associate flexibility with youth, when you feel flexible, you *feel* young. "Stiffness is one of the ways we perceive our age," says Bob Anderson of Palmer Lake, Colorado, author of *Stretching*. "Your flexibility influences how you see yourself and how you see your future. If you're stiff, you're losing contact with your body and your life.

"Stretching and flexibility help you avoid the muscular rigor mortis that is associated with aging," says Anderson.

When you're supple, you carry yourself the way you were meant to. "Flexibility helps correctly distribute your body weight over the bones and joints," says Dennis Humphrey, Ed.D., a professor in the biomedical sciences department at Southwest Missouri State University in Springfield. Appropriate weight distribution helps maintain correct posture. It also prevents individual muscles, joints and bones from being overburdened and makes them less susceptible to injury.

Working to retain—or regain—your flexibility now will help you as you get older. The problems many older people have in getting around are in part caused by inactivity in the past.

"Most people gradually stop being active," says Dr. Humphrey. "They stop challenging their joints, and consequently the joints become less flexible." The connective tissue that surrounds muscles also becomes stiffer, preventing adequate blood flow to muscles and joints. Deprived of oxygen, these muscles, connective tissues and joints become stiffer and decay.

Older people who have lost flexibility are predisposed to serious hip, leg and back injuries. "As you become less flexible in the back and hips, the tightening muscles and connective tissues cause your hips to slip forward and your back to arch," says Dr. Cornelius. "Not only does this throw off the entire range of motion in your lower body, it also causes your vertebrae to pinch the nerves in your back." That, in a nutshell, is how many older people lose mobility and eventually suffer severe back pain and injury.

## STRETCHING MAKES YOU SUPPLE

How do you limber up? By stretching. "Stretching is a muscle relaxer," says Dr. Cornelius. "It reduces the electrical activity, or nerve impulses, in the muscle, which in turn reduces muscle tension."

If you have had surgery recently or if you have any joint or muscle problems, you should consult your physician before you start a stretching program. Otherwise, you can forge ahead—gently. "Your body is very adaptable," says Dr. Humphrey. "But it doesn't like surprises. That means that when you start a flexibility program, you want to go very slowly. Don't make dramatic changes all at once. You need to be patient."

Don't force muscles to stretch; gently allow them to move into the tight zone, test the resistance and then relax. Each day, you can slightly increase the stretching of that tight zone. As you stretch, exhale; on the release, inhale. Wear loose clothing, and don't eat heavily before doing your stretching exercises.

If you run, ride an exercise bike or lift weights, you'll find that stretching is especially beneficial after a workout. It helps eliminate waste products produced by muscles during exercise and also reduces any muscle and joint trauma suffered during the workout. Dr. Humphrey, an expert in flexibility programs, recommends the following exercises.

**Reach for those toes.** Sit on the floor, your legs stretched out in front of you. Inhale, then reach as far as you can for your toes. As you stretch the backs of your legs, exhale. "Don't force it if it causes pain, and don't bounce," says Dr. Humphrey. Do this exercise slowly, allowing your back and the backs of your legs to stretch gently.

**Lift your legs.** While lying on your back, raise one leg so that it's perpendicular to the floor, with your knee straight. (Keep your other leg bent, with your foot on the floor.) Continue to move your leg toward your head, keeping your leg straight, while exhaling. Go as far as you can; relax. Do the same with the other leg. Repeat one or more times.

**Pull your legs in.** As you lie on your back, draw your legs toward your chest while wrapping your arms around them. Use your arms to pull your legs as close as you can into your stomach and chest, exhaling. Don't force the exercise. Repeat a couple of times.

**Rotate the trunk.** While sitting or standing, place your hands on your hips and rotate your trunk to the right as far as it will go. Exhale and push it a little farther. Now do it in the reverse direction.

**Stretch your thighs.** While standing, support your body by holding the wall with your right hand. Using your left hand, grab the back of your left ankle and pull it back toward your buttocks, stretching your thigh muscle. Do it slowly, exhaling. Alternate legs and repeat two or three times for each leg.

**Tilt your head.** While sitting or standing, tilt your head toward your shoulder. Do this on each side, left and right, allowing both sides of your neck to stretch, while exhaling. Do not allow your head to tip backward or forward, says Dr. Humphrey, because it can irritate or injure your spine.

**Twirl your feet.** While sitting on a chair, lift your leg and support it with a pillow so that your foot hangs freely above the floor. Rotate your foot in a counterclockwise direction. When your foot approaches the upper position, extend your toes upward so that your Achilles tendon and the bottom of your foot stretch. When your foot turns down, point your toes downward, stretching the top of your foot.

**Grip with your toes.** While sitting on a chair, place a towel on the floor in front of you and take off your shoes and socks. At the far end of the towel, place a 3- to 5-pound weight. At the near end, place your feet at the edge of the towel. Grip the towel with the toes of one foot and, using only the curling action of your toes, pull the towel and weight toward you. Repeat with the other foot.

## STRETCH ANYTIME, ANYWHERE

In addition to a regular stretching routine—or on the days you just don't have time to fit a session into your schedule—you can stretch throughout the day, even at your desk.

**Fight computer neck.** If you stare at a computer screen all day, you probably tend to poke your head out like a turtle. Get up once or twice a day, and stand or sit with your back flat against a wall. Pull your head back toward the wall and bring your chin down until it's tight. Repeat.

**Touch your back.** While seated, reach over your head to touch the back of your neck. Lower your arm to your side. Now reach behind you to touch the small of your back. Repeat ten times for both arms.

**Put your hands up.** Hold your hands over your head, palms together. Stretch your arms up and slightly backward.

**Shrug your shoulders.** While seated with your feet flat,

shrug your shoulders up and down. You could increase the stretch by holding a book in each hand as you shrug.

**Reach for it.** Every time you reach for something on a shelf, stretch gently as you reach.

---

### ANTI-AGING CHECKUP
## HOW FLEXIBLE ARE YOU?

Not sure if you're flexible enough or not? Dennis Humphrey, Ed.D., a professor in the biomedical sciences department at Southwest Missouri State University in Springfield, recommends three simple self-tests for determining if you have adequate range of motion and flexibility. Answer these questions Yes or No.

\_\_\_\_ Can you tie your shoes while in a sitting position without pain or discomfort?

\_\_\_\_ While standing, can you painlessly touch your toes without bending your knees or straining?

\_\_\_\_ Are you able to perform your normal daily activities without pain or discomfort?

#### INTERPRETING YOUR ANSWERS

If the answers to these questions are No, you may need to work on your flexibility, says Dr. Humphrey. For most people, the problem stems from a simple lack of flexibility. However, pain associated with movement can indicate a medical problem such as arthritis or heart disease and should be checked out by a doctor.

# 16

# FOOT PROBLEMS

### Relief for Painful or Tired Feet

**In** a normal day, each of your feet will hit the ground about 5,000 times; no matter what your weight, the cumulative impact on your feet is several hundred tons. And if you run or jump, that impact is tripled. During your lifetime, those feet will carry you about 150,000 miles—the equivalent of more than four trips around the world.

So it's no surprise that 75 percent of Americans complain of foot problems. It's a minor miracle that these wondrous workhorses we call feet endure their lifetime of pounding and punishment, especially in the less-than-perfect shoes we often wear.

### WHY OUR FEET COMPLAIN

We bring on some of our foot problems ourselves with shoes that are poorly designed or don't fit properly. More than half of all American women, for example, wear shoes that are at least one size too small, says Dean Wakefield, director of public affairs at the American Podiatric Medical Association in Bethesda, Maryland.

Also, more than 60 percent of women wear high heels, the most damaging type of shoe. High heels are designed to shift the body's weight to the front of the foot, where the toes are crammed into the tiny toe box. The toes, foot bones, ligaments and muscles are squeezed so tightly that circulation is restricted and pain is inevitable. The shoe's height and its unstable spiked heel stress the muscles and tendons of the foot and can cause multiple injuries.

In addition, simple aging and diseases such as diabetes, arthritis and circulatory disorders also lead to foot problems. "Nearly everyone has some kind of foot problem from time to time," notes Simon Nzuzi, D.P.M., podiatric medical director of the Foot Clinics of New York.

## KINDER, GENTLER SHOES

Thanks in large measure to major sports figures such as Larry Bird, Magic Johnson and Michael Jordan, the footwear industry has burgeoned in the past 15 years. Not only are there more sports shoes, there's a whole realm of walking shoes and more comfortable dress shoes. It's a development the American Podiatric Medical Association generally favors. "There's plenty of marketing glitz out there," Wakefield says, "but a lot of what is presented is based on good research." Here are some tips to help you select the shoes that are best for you.

**Ditch the stiletto heels.** Okay, most women won't give up their high heels completely, but whenever possible they should choose what Wakefield calls a walking pump. "The walking pump has a broader toe box, a broader reinforced heel, with a bigger surface area than the spike heel," he says. "The heel isn't as high as the spiked-heeled shoe, and the pump is better cushioned. But while it's a good development, it's not the ideal shoe."

**Shop in the afternoon.** Feet tend to swell as the day progresses. Therefore, shop for shoes later on, when your feet are a little larger and closer to their normal size.

**Check size carefully.** You want about a half-inch between your big toe and the front end of the shoe, and the heel of the shoe shouldn't slip up and down as you walk.

**Go for a good fit.** You've found the perfect pair of shoes, but they're just a bit, well, tight and painful. Don't assume that they'll get "broken in." Shoes generally don't change much—what will be broken in are your feet.

**Consider ventilation.** The 250,000 sweat glands in your feet can release more than 6 ounces of sweat per day. To keep your feet dry, shoes must allow proper ventilation. This means selecting materials such as leather or nylon mesh.

**Choose the right shoe for the sport.** Footwear that's right for one sport may be wrong for another. A shoe designed for a certain sport offers specialized cushioning and reinforced features that protect against damage due to the demands of that activity. "Tennis requires a lot of quick starts and stops, with bursts of speed," says Wakefield, "while jogging and aerobic dance require a very different range of motion from your feet and shoes."

## TLC FOR YOUR FEET

We all need a little extra love from time to time, and our feet are no different. Here are some ways to treat them right.

**Take a walk.** You might think that walking would tire your feet, but it's one of the best things you can do for them. Walking improves blood circulation, increases flexibility and helps keep bones and muscles toned and healthy.

**Raise your feet.** Whenever possible, elevate your feet and wiggle your toes to improve circulation and relax the muscles.

**Give a massage.** Gently rub your feet, or swap massages with a friend. Massage the whole foot while rotating your thumbs to promote circulation and relieve tense spots. Slide your thumb deeply along the arches. Use soothing oils occasionally.

**Stick your toes in the tub.** Soak your feet in warm water containing Epsom salts for 15 to 20 minutes—a time-honored home remedy that still revitalizes the feet and entire body.

## COPING WITH CORNS AND CALLUSES

Constant rubbing by shoes can cause protective layers of the skin to form. Corns are small areas of thickened skin on toes, often caused by pressure of a shoe. Calluses are broader patches of dead skin, usually located at the bottom of the foot and along the heel. Both corns and calluses can cause pain, especially if your shoe fits tightly and presses the hardened skin against a nerve or bone in the foot.

*Editor's note:* If you have diabetes or peripheral vascular disease, consult your physician about your special foot-care needs before attempting to remedy corns, calluses or other problems on your own.

**Have a soak.** The first step in treating corns and calluses is to soak your feet in warm water (never hot) to soften the skin.

**Rub them away.** Use a pumice stone or callus file to gently rub the corn or callus away from the skin. It may require several such treatments, but don't become so zealous that you rub the skin raw.

### BANISHING BUNIONS AND BUNIONETTES

Bunions, those swollen and misaligned joints leading to the big toe, are apt to appear anytime; bunionettes, the smaller versions, turn up at the joint leading to the fifth, or little, toe. They are ten times more common among women than men, primarily because women have more of a tendency to wear ill-fitting shoes. You can take steps to protect your toes.

**Choose your shoes carefully.** The most common and successful treatment for bunions is simply to wear shoes that fit properly, with plenty of room at the front. Rubber-soled, all-terrain sandals (such as those made by Nike and Teva), cork footbed sandals (such as Birkentocks) and properly fitting athletic shoes are ideal.

**Have your shoes stretched.** If necessary, shoemakers can stretch your shoes to provide greater comfort and movement to the front of the foot.

### ANNIHILATING ATHLETE'S FOOT

This fungal infection is encouraged by a lack of adequate ventilation, often due to snug and sweaty socks or shoes that are too tight. So keep your feet clean, dry and well ventilated. Here's how.

**Groom daily.** Wash your feet with soap and water daily and dry them thoroughly. (You can use a hair dryer on a low setting to blow-dry your feet.)

## ANTI-AGING CHECKUP
# POINTERS FOR HAPPY FEET

When your feet feel good, you feel good. Follow this check-list to help keep your feet healthy and strong. Do you:

____ Inspect your feet daily for cuts, abrasions, ingrown nails or calluses?

____ Have your feet examined by a doctor at least twice a year if you have diabetes or are over 50?

____ Bathe your feet daily? "Most of us wash everywhere else on our body, and if some soap falls on our feet we think we've washed our feet," says Dean Wakefield of the American Podiatric Medical Association. Our feet deserve better than that! Bathe your feet in warm water, not hot. Since people with diabetes may have lost some sensitivity in their feet, they should avoid hot water or surfaces that can burn their feet.

____ Keep your feet dry and warm?

____ Keep your toenails well trimmed and cut straight across?

____ Check your shoes for pebbles or other foreign objects before you put them on?

____ Do regular aerobic exercise, such as walking, bicycling or swimming, to promote circulation?

____ Take off your shoes from time to time during the day and sit with your feet raised whenever possible to improve circulation?

____ Wear clean socks and stockings?

____ Avoid clothing that will reduce circulation to the legs and feet, such as elastic waistbands, garter belts and stockings and socks that are too tight?

____ Stay away from cigarettes and smokers? Smoke causes atherosclerosis and reduces circulation.

### INTERPRETING YOUR ANSWERS

If you have foot problems that don't go away with home treatments, you should see a doctor. You should also seek medical care if foot pain persists, your feet hurt more as the
*continued*

---

day goes on, or discomfort keeps you from putting your shoe on or keeping them on. Another clue that it's time to see the doctor is if the first few steps of the day bring the most acute pain.

Whom do you see? Orthopedists treat all types of bone and muscle problems, and podiatrists treat foot problems. Both can do surgery and prescribe medical treatments. Dermatologists can treat rashes or athlete's foot. It's best to ask your primary doctor for a referral.

---

**Give your feet air.** Go barefoot and wear sandals when possible. And wear cotton-blend or acrylic socks that wick away moisture. Make sure your shoes are dry when you put them on, and rotate wearing several pairs so each has time to air out.

**Buy shower footwear.** Athlete's foot is contagious, so try to avoid walking barefoot in public showers. Use antifungal powder or ointment on your feet periodically, after any exposure.

### DEALING WITH OTHER FOOT PROBLEMS

Here are some easy solutions for some other common foot problems.

**Try OTCs for plantar warts.** These growths appear on the sole, or plantar, surface of the foot and usually disappear on their own within two years. Often they are painless, but those that put pressure on a nerve cause severe pain. Over-the-counter topical medications that include salicylic acid are usually successful in getting rid of the wart. If the medication doesn't work, see a podiatrist, but never try to cut off the wart yourself.

**Protect blisters.** It's best not to pop a blister, as that bubble of skin provides a protective layer. Put moleskin or an adhesive bandage on it, and wear socks to help protect the blister. If it breaks on its own, apply an antiseptic and a bandage or a product called 2nd Skin. This dressing is moist and will help protect the skin underneath.

If a blister will burst from the pressure of walking, wash the area, then make a small hole near the edge with a needle you've sterilized in a flame or alcohol. Gently squeeze out the liquid.

**Relieve ingrown toenails.** These are often painful and can become infected. Tight shoes and improperly trimmed toenails are the most common causes—the nail of the big toe presses into the toe's soft tissue. Trim your toenails straight across, leaving a margin at the edges. File any sharp edges with an emery board; never tear the nail with your fingers.

To treat an ingrown toenail, podiatrists suggest you soak your foot in warm or cool water to soften the nail. Dry carefully, then place small wads of cotton under the toenail to relieve the pressure on the soft tissue while the nail grows out. Replace the cotton wads several times a day if necessary. Wear open-toed shoes if possible, and consult a physician if the problem persists or the toe becomes infected.

**Heed heel pain.** Heel spurs are calcium deposits that can form at the heel or underside of the foot. They may result from arthritis, lack of circulation in the feet or shoes that do not adequately support the heel. Both heel pain and spurs are associated with the inflammation of the connective tissue that runs from the heel to the ball of the foot. The pain usually disappears by itself, without treatment, but if it persists, consult a physician.

**Fight foot odor.** First, change your socks frequently, more than once a day if necessary. Wear 100 percent cotton socks or socks made of wicking material, such as Thor-Lo or Coolmax. Also, never wear the same pair of shoes two days in a row; they need at least 24 hours to dry out between wearings. If these changes don't help, try antiperspirants or commercial foot powders, or soak your feet in a mixture of vinegar and water.

# 17

# GALLSTONES

You *Can* Avoid These Pesky Stones

**You** probably never even think about your gallbladder. Until it acts up, that is. Each year, some 500,000 Americans have their gallbladders removed, and more than a million others discover that they have gallstones.

So what exactly is this troublesome little organ? It's a small, pear-shaped sac on the right side of your body, right behind your liver. The gallbladder stores bile, an acid-rich substance produced by the liver to help digest fats, and secretes it into the intestines when needed.

Normally, the bile acids in the gallbladder keep both cholesterol and calcium in solution form. But when there's too much cholesterol in the bile or not enough of the substances that help keep things in solution, some of the contents may crystallize into stones.

Eight out of ten gallstones are composed primarily of cholesterol; the others are made up of bile pigments and calcium. The stones themselves can be as small as a grain of sand or as large as an egg, and they can form in either the gallbladder or the bile ducts that connect the gallbladder and liver to the small intestine.

Half of those with gallstones don't even know they have them because the stones do not cause any problems. When a stone gets lodged in a duct leading from the gallbladder to the small intestine, however, the pain can be severe and excruciatingly prolonged, lasting anywhere from 20 minutes to several hours. More often than not, the gallbladder has to be removed.

Women between the ages of 20 and 60 are three times more likely to develop gallstones than men in the same age-group, but by the time men and women reach their 60s, the rate of gallstones is roughly equal. Scientists suspect one reason more young women get gallstones than men is that the female hormone estrogen causes higher levels of cholesterol to accumulate within the bile. Also, oral contraceptives and estrogen replacement therapy, being overweight, going on crash diets or eating a high-fat, low-fiber diet can contribute to gallstones.

## TO AVOID GALLSTONES, CHANGE YOUR DIET

The comforting news about gallstones is that if you don't have them now, you can avoid them. Here's how.

**Add fiber and cut back on fat.** Cultures that routinely consume high-fat, low-fiber diets—such as people in the United States, Great Britain and Sweden—suffer more gallstones than those who eat high-fiber, low-fat diets, as many Asians do. When Asians migrate to the United States and adopt typical American eating patterns, however, their rates of gallstones go up sixfold within a single generation.

You can spare yourself gallstones by lowering the fat content of your diet and boosting your fiber intake. That means not eating as many animal foods and eating more whole grains, vegetables and fruit.

**Take off excess pounds.** A study conducted by the Harvard School of Public Health followed 88,837 women over four years and found that *all* the women who had their gallbladders removed were overweight. "Overall, we observed a roughly linear relationship between relative weight and the risk of gallstones," reported the researchers in the *New England Journal of Medicine*. Even being moderately overweight raised the risk, the researchers found, but seriously obese women had six times the risk of suffering gallstones as women who were not overweight. (For tips on losing weight, see chapter 27.)

**Cut back on cholesterol intake.** A study at Johns Hopkins University in Baltimore found that prairie dogs who were fed large amounts of cholesterol soon began to develop gallstones. While this doesn't necessarily mean that the same thing would happen in people, it *could*—and cutting cholesterol can lower your risks of high blood pressure, stroke and heart attack as well.

**Chow down on veggies.** Women in Athens, Greece, who developed gallstones ate relatively high quantities of starchy foods—such as pasta, rice, bread and potatoes—which is fine. But they didn't get enough vegetables, according to a study conducted by the University of Massachusetts School of Public Health. In fact, the researchers found that "a modest protective effect was observed among women reporting relatively high consumption of vegetables of all kinds."

**Don't skip meals.** People who wait as long as 16 hours between meals—and that includes the time span between supper and the next day's breakfast—may increase their risk of gallstones. A study published in the *American Journal of Public Health* reported that the amount of cholesterol in the bile of women with gallbladder disease increased as the time between meals lengthened, rising 12-fold at the 16-hour point. And high cholesterol in the bile contributes to the formation of gallstones.

**Eat frequent, high-fiber meals.** Your best bet to avoid gallstones, say scientists, is to eat frequent meals consisting of lots of vegetables, grains and fruit.

## DEALING WITH TROUBLESOME GALLSTONES

Once you have gallstones that are acting up, the most common medical solution is removing the gallbladder—an organ that, like the appendix, you can easily do without, say doctors. Without the gallbladder, the bile just goes straight from the liver to the small intestine. In some cases, the stones can be dissolved without resorting to surgery. Here's the lowdown on medical tactics against gallstones.

**Dissolve those stones.** Oral drugs that increase bile acids and dissolve stones are most effective against small stones, 5 to 20 millimeters in diameter (the size of a penny), and when used in conjunction with a low-fat, low-cholesterol diet. These drugs are also more effective for people who are not overweight. Dissolving the stones can take six months to two years of treatment, so this is no quick fix.

**Shock-wave them away.** Another common therapy is extracorporeal shock-wave lithotripsy, the bombardment of the gallstones by ultrasonic waves. This technique can only be used, however, on gallbladders that contain no more than three stones no larger than 30 millimeters in diameter each (about the size of a quarter).

**Consider a new kind of surgery.** Finally, a new procedure called a laparoscopic cholescystectomy can remove the gallbladder without the 4- to 6-inch abdominal incision required by traditional operations. A long tube, equipped with a tiny video camera at the end, is inserted through the navel and guided into the gallbladder area. Three small incisions are made in the abdomen to allow probelike instruments to remove the stones and the bile. The gallbladder itself is then removed through the hole in the navel. While conventional gallbladder surgery requires six days of recovery, the new procedure allows patients to get up and move around immediately after surgery and requires only an overnight hospital stay.

---

**ANTI-AGING CHECKUP**
## SIGNS OF A PESKY GALLBLADDER

Not every sharp pain in the solar plexus signals gallbladder trouble. Conversely, you can have gallstones without experiencing any symptoms. Below is a checklist of factors that increase the likelihood of the disease. Only your doctor can tell you for sure if you have gallstones, but you should seek medical advice if you check off any of the last three signs listed.

_____ You are overweight. You are especially at risk if you are 20 percent or more over your ideal weight.

_____ You are also female or of Native American or Mexican-American descent.

_____ You suffer from chronic indigestion, nausea, vomiting or belching. These symptoms may indicate that stones are growing inside the gallbladder.

_____ You have experienced severe abdominal pain or jaundice (yellow skin and eyeballs). This can be caused by stones blocking the bile duct.

*continued*

_____ You have suffered one or more confirmed gallbladder attacks. Gallstone symptoms can come and go, but once
you have had one, you are likely to have another.

## INTERPRETING YOUR ANSWERS

A typical gallbladder attack is pain in the upper-right quadrant of your body that radiates around to the back or right
shoulder blade. The pain is sharp and stabbing, rather than a
dull, constant pressure. It may be brought on by eating a meal,
particularly a high-fat one. In contrast, ulcer or gastritis pain
occurs under the sternum or mid-abdomen, and it's burning
and persistent. Ulcer pain may be relieved rather than worsened by eating.

# 18

# HEARING

### Take Steps *Now* to Preserve
### This Vital Sense

**Just** listening to music or the soft words of love can lift the soul to heavenly heights. But those with serious hearing problems may never know that joy. For anyone who suffers from profound hearing loss or the internal racket of tinnitus, the inner world can be a prison of frustrating silence or a siege of ceaseless noise.

Nearly 20 million Americans suffer from some degree of actual hearing loss, and another 40 to 50 million suffer from tinnitus, an ongoing array of inner-ear noise that can range from a low-level hum to a loud and destabilizing buzz, ringing or roar. For some, the two problems overlay: As hearing dims, annoying interior noises emerge from the silence.

Most people with hearing loss are over age 50, but a significant number are only in their 30s and 40s, thanks in part to being bombarded with loud music during their teens and early 20s. (Many rock artists themselves are quite hard of hearing.) Tinnitus, on the other hand, can occur at any age, from childhood to senior years. We'll look at both of these problems and investigate the treatments available. But first, let's explore steps that can be taken to keep our hearing in the first place.

## MAKE YOUR HEARING LAST

Listening to Led Zeppelin at top volume isn't the only thing that can impair your hearing. So can mowing the lawn or using a jackhammer without protection, or getting an infection or injury to one or more of the tiny organs that make up your hearing apparatus. The result may range from minor impairment to total deafness. In any case, it's never too late to protect (or improve) your hearing.

**Take care with your eardrums.** Never poke any sharp object—a matchstick, paper clip or bobby pin—into your ear. Puncturing the eardrum can prevent sound from being transferred to the inner ear. Often a puncture heals on its own, but in severe cases surgery may be needed to restore hearing.

**Let earwax take care of itself.** You may commonly use swabs or other items to try to remove earwax, but it's not a good idea. Usually, these "aids" only push the wax deeper into the ear, forcing it against the eardrum. Normally, dried or accumulated wax falls out of the ear and is easily washed away.

**For problem wax, reach for a solution.** Sometimes hearing loss is simply due to nature's overdoing things. Wax can build up inside the ear canal, obstructing the passage of sound waves to the inner ear.

We all *need* to protect our inner ears from insects, bacteria and dust, repel water and help ward off infections of the ear canal, but it should not accumulate. Once your doctor has confirmed that the problem is excessive or packed earwax, you can remove the wax with over-the-counter or prescription medications.

## Avoid Big Bangs

A more serious impairment can result from an injury to the inner ear or cochlea, where thousands of tiny hairs transform vibration into nerve impulses that travel along the auditory nerve to the brain. This area can be damaged by excessively loud noise—jet takeoffs, gunshots or highly amplified rock music.

"Compared to their parents, today's young people are at a significantly increased risk of noise-related hearing loss due to Walkman-type earphone radios played at high volume, highly amplified rock concerts and other modern business and leisure equipment," cautions Charles W. Parkins, M.D., professor of otolaryngology at Louisiana State University Medical Center in New Orleans. Here's what you can do to help preserve your hearing.

**Lower the volume.** Some household appliances produce constant sound that can traumatize the nerves of the inner ear, making them less and less responsive, until the nerves finally die off. Continuous noise over a long period can be more damaging to the ear than intermittent sounds. This is true even though we may no longer even notice the ongoing noise.

Reduce the volume by placing foam pads under machines such as food processors and surrounding dishwashers with sound-deadening material. Put your computer printer in a sound-reducing box. Install sound-absorbing carpeting and draperies in noisy rooms. Shop for the quietest products available when purchasing items such as lawn mowers, air conditioners and leaf blowers.

**Muff your ears.** Jets, power tools, loud music, traffic, target ranges and subways all produce enough noise to be dangerous, especially for those who must endure them on a regular basis. Buy a pair of special sound-reducing earmuffs (sold in sporting goods stores and catalogs) or earplugs so you can shut out the noise. They aren't expensive, and if you already have some degree of hearing loss, they can fend off further deficiencies. Choose muffs with a noise-reduction rating of at least 20.

**Have your hearing checked.** Regular testing can detect small losses of hearing and offer corrective action before more noticeable losses show up—such as the inability to hear parts of a conversation. Specialists use a device called an audiometer that generates tones of various frequencies. The test is done quickly—it only takes 30 minutes or so—and can accurately determine the site and cause of hearing loss. Once an accurate diagnosis is made, treatment of the underlying disorder can commence. Your family doctor can help you find a physician to administer the test.

## QUIETING THE BUZZ OF TINNITUS

For most people with tinnitus, the inner buzzing, ringing or rumbling is so subtle that it goes unnoticed most of the time. The lucky ones experience the condition for only a few hours or a few days, and then it disappears. But for about 12 million people, tinnitus is both severe and disruptive to their lives. The best thing is to seek help.

## HEARING AIDS ARE BETTER THAN EVER

Hearing aids have come a long way over the years.

"There have been tremendous advances in our knowledge about how to improve hearing with aids and with the design, technology and fitting of such aids," says Lawrence M. Posen, president of Beltone Electronics Corporation, the largest U.S. manufacturer of hearing aids and hearing testing equipment.

In the past, hearing aids amplified *all* sound equally, while the wearer might hear perfectly well in certain ranges. "Now, to compensate for each individual's specific hearing loss, we can customize the aid by adjusting the shape of the frequency response," says Posen. This ability to amplify sound selectively prevents you from being blasted in ranges where you have little or no hearing loss.

"If you're walking through a busy airport, for example, and you can still hear your tinnitus despite all the racket, it's probably interfering with your life," says Jack Vernon, Ph.D., professor of otolaryngology at the Oregon Hearing Research Center at Oregon Health Sciences University in Portland. "And that's when you should see a doctor."

Unfortunately, the cause of tinnitus often eludes physicians, causing considerable frustration in the patient. "Treatment tends to be a matter of trial and error," says Steven Berman, Ph.D., assistant professor and director of audiology at the Medical College of Pennsylvania in Philadelphia. "What works for one person may not work for others." But physicians can usually help relieve symptoms, if not cure the problem. Here are some treatment options.

## ANTI-AGING CHECKUP
# A WRITTEN HEARING TEST

The following simple test will help you determine if you have a hearing loss and should see an ear, nose and throat (E.N.T.) specialist. Respond to the following statements, using any of the four possible answers given below. Note the respective points associated with each response, and total your points after you finish.

Almost always: 3 points
Half the time: 2 points
Occasionally: 1 point
Never: 0 points

_____  1. I have a problem hearing over the telephone.

_____  2. It's hard for me to follow the conversation when two or more people are talking at the same time.

_____  3. People complain that I turn the TV volume up too high.

_____  4. I have to strain to understand conversations.

_____  5. I sometimes don't hear common sounds, such as the phone or doorbell ringing.

_____  6. Hearing conversations when there's a noisy background, such as at a party, is a problem for me.

_____  7. I get confused about where the sounds I hear come from.

_____  8. I misunderstand some words in a sentence and need to ask people to repeat themselves.

_____  9. The speech of women and children is especially hard for me to understand.

_____ 10. I have worked in noisy environments (such as in assembly lines or around jackhammers or jet engines).

_____ 11. Many people I talk to seem to be mumbling or not speaking clearly.

_____ 12. People get annoyed because I misunderstand what they say.

*continued*

_____ 13. I misunderstand what others are saying and make inappropriate responses.

_____ 14. Because I cannot hear well and fear that I might reply improperly, I avoid social activities.

_____ 15. Ask a family member or friend to answer this question: Do you think this person has a hearing loss?

**Total:** ——

### INTERPRETING YOUR ANSWERS

*0 to 5:* Your hearing is probably fine. No further tests are required.

*6 to 9:* Seeing an E.N.T. specialist is suggested.

*10 and above:* Seeing an E.N.T. specialist is strongly recommended.

SOURCE: Reprinted by permission of the *Johns Hopkins Medical Letter Health after 50*. Copyright © Medletter Associates, 1991.

**Clear up medical problems.** "Tinnitus can be a symptom of several other possible disorders," says Dr. Berman. It might signal an infection of the inner ear, a partially blocked artery or an autoimmune disorder. Simply treating the underlying disorder successfully usually eliminates the tinnitus.

**Treat your allergies.** Ragweed, pollen, mold and other common airborne allergens or troublesome foods are among the underlying causes of tinnitus, according to Ronald G. Amedee, M.D., assistant professor of otolaryngology at Tulane Medical Center in New Orleans. "With proper treatment of allergies, you may be able to at least control your level of tinnitus or eliminate it entirely," he says. Some people notice improvement after eliminating dairy products and other foods that may cause allergic reactions. Other sufferers are helped by seeking treatment for ragweed, pollen and mold allergies.

**Check out the "Gang of Five."** Possible culprits also include aspirin, quinine, nicotine, alcohol, and caffeine. In high doses, aspirin and aspirin-containing remedies can induce temporary tinnitus or aggravate a permanent case, as can quinine and nicotine. Also, alcohol and caffeine aggravate tinnitus in some people. You may want to experiment with cutting back on these—one at a time—and see if your condition improves.

**Lower your blood pressure.** Circulatory disorders, particularly high blood pressure, which can raise the sound of one's heartbeat in the inner ear, can also contribute to tinnitus. A low-fat, low-salt diet, coupled with moderate exercise, works for some with tinnitus. (See chapter 6.)

**Drown out the drone.** You can also use a device that *masks* the underlying noise of tinnitus by overlapping it with another sound. Such hearing-aid-like pieces are inserted into the ear canal and emit a sound that, because it is external, is easier to accept and ignore. An ear, nose and throat specialist can help you choose from a variety of such sounds.

**Consider a hearing aid.** "About 95 percent of patients with tinnitus have some degree of hearing loss," says Dr. John House, M.D., associate clinical professor of otolaryngology at the University of Southern California School of Medicine in Los Angeles and president of the House Ear Institute. "Wearing a hearing aid can't get rid of the ringing, but the tinnitus may become less obvious if you can hear better."

**Ask your doctor about coping techniques.** For some people, learning to control the noise through biofeedback techniques, relaxation techniques or hypnosis works, says Dr. Berman. If your doctor is not trained in these, ask him or her to refer you to a practitioner experienced in such techniques.

**Reach out for emotional help.** Because tinnitus can be so frustrating, many who have it also suffer emotionally, especially from depression. All the experts recommend getting help to cope with any emotional repercussions from tinnitus. Maybe all you need is some daily exercise to ease frustration. Otherwise, counseling or better coping techniques may help.

Many local support groups for tinnitus sufferers meet regularly to share information and coping mechanisms. You can find such a self-help group in your area by writing to the American Tinnitus Association, P.O. Box 5, Portland, OR 97207.

# 19

# HEART DISEASE

Not Necessarily the American Way

**Don't** let heart disease intimidate you. Dealing with it is like negotiating highway traffic: Both are risky, and there are plenty of alarming statistics that tell you all that can go wrong. But if you're smart, you do all you can to protect yourself and make sure everything goes right!

Before you hit the highway, you check your car for safety—brakes, tires, lights. Then you resolve to drive sober, heed the speed limit, drive defensively and stop if you get sleepy. These reasonable precautions make you feel secure. You know you've greatly reduced the chances you'll have an accident.

Take the same approach to heart disease, and it may never touch you. Even if you already have heart disease, the good news is that it can be cured—often without medication.

To achieve your goals, you must be willing to take reasonable precautions that may include changing lifestyle patterns that are the very cause of the illness.

### CLOGGING CAN'T CONTINUE WITHOUT CONSEQUENCES

The underlying cause of most of the heart disease that afflicts nearly 70 million Americans is atherosclerosis, or cholesterol plaques that clog the coronary arteries leading to the heart, according to the American Heart Association. These plaques interfere with blood flow to the heart. Ultimately, they can stop blood and oxygen from reaching the heart entirely—resulting in a heart attack.

The extent of clogging is directly proportional to the amount of cholesterol in the bloodstream, especially low density lipoproteins, or LDLs. On the other hand, high density lipoproteins (HDLs) protect against the damaging effects of LDLs and against heart disease. What's both exciting and encouraging is that we can control the amount as well as the type of cholesterol in our bloodstream.

You can help lower your cholesterol levels by reducing the amount of fat and meat in your diet, increasing your intake of vegetables and other high-fiber foods, getting plenty of vitamin C and exercising regularly. (See chapter 8.)

## A DOZEN AND ONE WAYS TO SAVE YOUR HEART

By now, your confidence should be way up! You really do have the power to protect yourself. Here are more than a dozen ways to beat heart disease, based on the advice of leading experts.

**Clear the smoke to brighten your future.** Good news: Cigarette smokers can dramatically reduce their health risks simply by stopping the habit, according to researchers at Harvard Medical School. Think of this—if 25 percent of the nation's cigarette smokers quit today, there would be at least 415,000 fewer cases of heart disease by the year 2015! The best advice: If you smoke, stop; if you don't, never start.

The problem is that cigarette smoking raises your blood levels of both LDL and triglycerides (harmful fatty acids that also contribute to heart disease) and drive down your HDL levels. These all put you at risk for heart attack or stroke.

And cigarette smoking causes blood clots, the underlying cause of 90 percent of all heart attacks, according to the American Heart Association. People who smoke are 20 times more likely to die of heart disease than nonsmokers who don't have cholesterol and blood pressure concerns. In 1989, cigarette smoking was directly responsible for 115,000 deaths from heart disease.

**High blood pressure is a red flag.** When high blood pressure or hypertension is in the picture, there's a greater likelihood of cardiovascular diseases, including heart attack and stroke. Hypertension has no obvious symptoms, so regular blood pressure checks are a must, especially if heart disease is part of the family history. (See chapter 6 on good blood pressure control.)

**Exercise does a body good.** Regular aerobic exercise, such as 20 to 30 minutes of brisk walking, three or four times a week, will raise your HDLs and lower your LDLs, according to a study published in the *Journal of the American Medical Association.* Not only will this reduce your risk of heart disease significantly, but exercise adds to the oxygen in all the muscles in your body, including your heart. That makes your heart's job—pumping oxygen-laden blood throughout the body—much easier. Exercise also makes your heart more efficient, causing it to pump more blood per beat while increasing the time it rests between beats.

Even a little exercise goes a very long way. "You receive the optimal benefits by working out 20 minutes a day, five days a week, at your target heart rate," says Thomas Kottke, M.D., a cardiologist at the Mayo Clinic in Rochester, Minnesota. "But the message has been confused. People think they won't get anything out of it if they do less. While a brisk walk 20 minutes a day would make a major impact, the population, on the average, is so sedentary that any exercise other than changing TV channels or cracking a beer is great." (See chapter 1 for more about exercise.)

**Drop the saturated-fat foods.** Since elevated blood cholesterol is the basis for most heart disease, experts recommend that we reduce our intake of the source of the problem—dietary saturated fat and cholesterol. That means animal foods, such as red meat, chicken, eggs and whole dairy products. A few plant foods, such as coconuts, avocados and palm oils, also contain saturated fat, but most vegetables and all whole grains contain the more healthful monounsaturated and polyunsaturated oils.

While saturated fat dramatically elevates your cholesterol level, particularly your LDLs, mono- and polyunsaturated fats lower LDLs and elevate HDLs. Therefore, cardiologists recommend that we select whole grains, vegetables and nuts, all of which contain the cholesterol-lowering fats. Many white-fish, shellfish and salmon contain a type of polyunsaturated oil called omega-3 that also cuts cholesterol.

Whole grains, vegetables and fruits also provide soluble fiber, which binds with LDLs and helps eliminate them from the body. Oats, oat bran, brown rice, citrus fruits and most legumes (peas, beans, lentils) are good sources of soluble fiber.

**Curtail cholesterol, too.** Only animal foods contain dietary cholesterol, which most Americans consume at the rate of about 500 milligrams per day. Because dietary cholesterol elevates blood cholesterol, the American Heart Association recommends that we reduce our intake to 300 milligrams. Cutting down on animal food means consuming less saturated fat, thereby lowering blood cholesterol levels.

**It's better to trim all fat.** Reduce *all* dietary fats, says William Castelli, M.D., director of the famed Framingham Heart Study, a long-term study gathering health-related data on the adult residents of Framingham, Massachusetts. "If you reduce all dietary fat, you automatically knock down saturated-fat intake because about half of the fat we eat is saturated," he says.

This is especially important if you are overweight. A teaspoon of fat—even vegetable fat—contains twice the calories of a teaspoon of carbohydrate. That's why it's almost impossible to lose weight on a high-fat diet.

**Consider aspirin.** Aspirin helps prevent the blood from clotting and thereby protects against the most common cause of heart attacks. Dr. Castelli says that taking regular doses of aspirin is probably a good idea if you fall into one of the following high-risk groups: those who have already had a heart attack; all men over 50; men over 40 with a family history of heart disease; those with uncontrollable high blood pressure or a high cholesterol level; or people with diabetes.

Typically, doctors recommend 160 milligrams of aspirin daily, or half a standard aspirin, according to George Sopko, M.D., a cardiologist at the National Heart, Lung and Blood Institute in Bethesda, Maryland. However, Dr. Sopko advises consulting a physician before taking regular doses of aspirin. Some people experience undesirable side effects, including ulcers.

**Keep your weight down.** The more you weigh, the harder your heart must work to pump blood through your body. New research suggests that overweight may be even harder on younger hearts than older ones. One study reported in the *American Journal of Cardiology* showed that obese men age 45 and younger had three times more incidence of hypertension than older men who were also overweight. Hypertension is a leading risk factor in heart attack and stroke, so keeping your weight level where it belongs could be your heart's salvation.

**Watch your cholesterol level.** Getting your cholesterol level checked is among the best ways of knowing whether your heart is at risk. "People have heard the message about heart disease and fat," says Dr. Kottke, "but they're not inclined to take advice until they think, 'Hey, that's me.' "

In addition to knowing your overall cholesterol level, you should know your HDL, LDL and triglyceride numbers, too. According to Robert Rosenson, M.D., director of the lipoprotein laboratory and co-director of preventive cardiology at Rush Presbyterian Hospital in Chicago, people with a healthy heart should have an LDL of just under 130 mg/dl (milligrams per deciliter of blood), while those with heart disease should expect that number to be less than 100. Triglycerides should be under 150 mg/dl, and people should shoot for an HDL of 50 and above.

**Nourish your heart with antioxidants.** Antioxidant vitamins A, C and E may slow or even prevent an oxidation process that is the underlying cause of heart disease, says Daniel Steinberg, M.D., professor of medicine at the University of California, San Diego. Scientists believe that atherosclerosis forms when white blood cells gobble up LDL in the bloodstream. Once the white cells become laden with LDL, they become part of the artery wall, where they oxidize and form cholesterol plaques. These vitamins, however, can apparently halt the oxidation.

Two studies at Harvard Medical School offer support to this theory. Women who took in 208 international units (I.U.) of vitamin E daily had much lower chances of having heart disease as those who had only 2.8 I.U. per day. (The recommended dietary allowance is 12 to 15 I.U. per day.) Similar results were found for men.

Foods that are rich in antioxidants include many whole

grains, fresh vegetables and fruit. (For more about antioxidants, see chapters 8 and 25.)

**Be sure to get your B vitamins.** Whole grains, vegetables and fruits are also good sources of the B vitamins, including folate and $B_6$. These nutrients may help combat homocysteine, a heart-threatening amino acid combination in the blood. Homocysteine is normally formed by the body but seldom accumulates to excessive levels because the B vitamins keep it in check. When the level rises (in an estimated 5 to 10 percent of the population), the cause is either genetic weakness or a shortage of the necessary B vitamins.

A study by Paul F. Jacques, Sc.D., assistant professor at the School of Nutrition at Tufts University, U.S. Department of Agriculture Human Nutrition Research Center on Aging, Boston, suggests that high homocysteine levels might explain heart attacks in people with no apparent risk factors. Doctors stop short of recommending universal supplements of folate for protection against heart disease, but there's no reason not to ensure sufficient folate intake by eating plenty of B-rich foods.

**Pay attention to your personal life.** Learning to enjoy love and friendship ranks above controlling the salt shaker and choosing decaf coffee over regular as a heart preserver, according to 200 heart experts. Sixty-four percent classified the positive influences of love on cardiovascular health as important, very important or extremely important. More than half felt that avoiding hostility—especially if you are hypertensive—or type-A behavior is important.

Finally, 40 percent of these doctors urged people to deal effectively with stress. Stress has been shown to weaken the immune system and to have an adverse effect on both hormone and cholesterol levels. Prayer, meditation and exercise are all known to reduce stress, improve cholesterol levels and balance hormones.

**Your heart responds to hormones.** If you are a postmenopausal woman, hormone replacement therapy could be a primary means of protecting your heart. We know that estrogen elevates HDL and decreases LDL levels, lowers blood pressure and lowers weight. Scientists also have evidence that estrogen lowers the incidence of heart disease among women.

That's especially important because heart disease is the leading cause of death among women.

Hormone therapy may slightly raise your risk of contracting breast cancer and is not recommended if, for instance, breast cancer runs in your family. Discuss hormone therapy with your doctor to determine if it's right for you.

---

### ANTI-AGING CHECKUP
## SIGNS OF HEART PROBLEMS

While there's no hard-and-fast way of predicting who will suffer heart problems, this quick quiz will give you an idea of whether or not you're at risk. Answer Yes or No to each question.

_____ Are you more than 20 pounds overweight?

_____ Do you have a family history of heart disease?

_____ Do you smoke or live with a person who smokes in the house?

_____ Are you sedentary and exercise only rarely?

_____ Are your triglyceride levels higher than 150 mg/dl?

_____ Do you often eat high-fat foods such as fried foods, butter, ice cream, sour cream and cheese?

_____ Is the ratio of your total cholesterol level to your HDL level more than 3.5 to 1?

_____ If you are around 60 years old, is your blood pressure consistently higher than 140/90?

_____ Do you feel that you're under a great deal of stress?

### INTERPRETING YOUR ANSWERS

If you answer Yes to more than one of these questions, you will probably want to check with your doctor and consider adopting some of the heart-disease-proofing measures presented in this chapter.

# 20

# IMMUNITY

### Double Your Immune Power

**You** can't see it, but chances are your immune system is at work right now, wiping out armies of bacteria and viruses that can cause all sorts of ailments. Every day, your defense system fights off disease and infection. Like an invisible shield against invisible predators, a healthy immune system enables you to:

- escape "nuisance" ailments such as sore throats, colds and the flu;
- travel to foreign lands without getting sick (well, usually);
- heal quickly after a cut, scrape or burn;
- minimize damage from pesticides or other toxins that accidentally make their way into the air or water supply;
- resist serious diseases, such as heart disease and cancer.

### REVITALIZE YOUR DEFENSES

About three out of four people find that, as they age, they're slightly more susceptible to "whatever's going around." Apparently, that's unnecessary: By improving nutrition and taking good care of your body's natural defenses, your immune system can remain healthy even as you grow older. Here are some ways to bolster your defense system.

**Eat well.** One of the tastiest and easiest ways to improve your immune system is to load up with the right groceries.

"The best advice is to eat the healthiest diet you can—one emphasizing fruits, vegetables and grains," says William Pryor, Ph.D., professor of chemistry and biochemistry and director of the Biodynamics Institute at Louisiana State University in Baton Rouge.

These foods contain nutrients—particularly beta-carotene and vitamins C and E—that have been shown to help fight diseases. These powerful nutrients are known as antioxidants and help battle the effect of free radicals, unstable molecules in your body. "We used to think that the effects of antioxidants were small," says Dr. Pryor. "Now we're finding that the effects are quite potent."

Also, vitamin C stimulates production of interferon, a substance that prevents viruses from taking hold, and helps keep white blood cells healthy. Vitamin E simulates the production of "killer" cells that seek out and destroy viruses, bacteria and cancer cells, says Ronald Ross Watson, Ph.D., an immunologist at the University of Arizona School of Medicine in Tucson. Beta-carotene stimulates macrophage cells—white blood cells that patrol your bloodstream and can produce chemicals that can kill cancer cells.

**Consider a supplement.** Even small additional amounts of certain nutrients can boost immune power, according to a study involving 96 people age 66 and older. One group received a supplement with moderate amounts of 18 nutrients, while the others received a pill similar in appearance but with only calcium and magnesium. The folks who got the 18 nutrients had fewer infections and only 23 sick days that year, while the other group had 48 sick days. Blood tests showed that the supplemented group had stronger immune systems, with more immune cells and a stronger immune response to viruses.

Roughly one-third of the group was low in some nutrients when the study started, which isn't uncommon in older folks. "For most people, you'd like to bolster the diet naturally with healthy foods like fruits and vegetables," says Ranjit Kumar Chandra, M.D., university research professor at Memorial University of Newfoundland and director of the World Health Organization Center for Nutritional Immunology. But if that's difficult or impossible, a balanced supplement would be the answer, he says.

The supplements in this study contained approximately the Recommended Dietary Allowance (RDA) levels of iron, zinc, copper, selenium, iodine, calcium, magnesium, vitamins A, C and D and the B vitamins, plus extra beta-carotene and vitamin E. If you choose to take a supplement, reach for a balanced vitamin and mineral supplement that doesn't exceed 100 percent of the RDA, say experts.

**Learn to manage stress.** The evidence is in: Stress *does* make you more susceptible to colds. In a landmark study, researchers gave cold viruses in nasal drops to 400 volunteers, while 26 people received drops without the cold virus. It turned out that the people who were identified as the most stressed were twice as likely to get colds as the others.

"Stress may stimulate hormones that help suppress the function of immune systems," says Redford B. Williams, M.D., professor of psychiatry and director of the Behavioral Medicine Research Center at Duke University Medical Center in Durham, North Carolina. "Helping people cope with stress may not just reduce infections, but research indicated it may also lower risks for heart disease." (See chapter 59 for more on stress.)

**Get a move on.** Moderate exercise stimulates the activity of immune cells and makes your whole immune system work better, concludes a report in *Sports Science Review*. Studies have shown that moderate exercise improves the ability of macrophage cells to wipe out invaders, including cancer cells. Also, moderate exercise is associated with fewer occurrences of colon, prostate and breast cancers. ("Moderate" means at least 30 minutes of aerobic exercise, such as walking or bicycling, three to five times a week.)

**Catch plenty of Zs.** During sleep, your body slows down certain activities and even shuts down others so it can devote itself to healing. When you're feeling ill or run down, a good night's sleep will help rebuild your defenses.

**Hide out from free radicals.** Free radicals are the unstable molecules that form the basis of many major diseases. Some free radicals result naturally from reactions within your body, but still more come from inhaling smoke, eating a fatty diet and being exposed to the untraviolet rays of the sun. Three easy steps to reduce exposure to free radicals:

- If you smoke, quit. (If you don't smoke, avoid breathing in smoke from other people.)
- Reduce fat in your diet. (See chapter 25 for fat-cutting tips.)
- Protect your skin from the sun with clothing and sun-screens—and by avoiding peak sunlight hours (usually 11:00 A.M. to 2:00 P.M.) whenever possible.

**Get a flu vaccination.** Research suggests that flu shots not only prevent viral flu infections but, if taken yearly, can also power up the immune system. When a group of adults in their 70s were given a flu vaccine, their declining immune systems were so bolstered that they matched those of a group of young adults. The vaccinated people were resistant against not only the particular flu strains in the vaccine but other strains as well, says Janet E. McElhaney, M.D., assistant professor of medicine at the University of Alberta in Edmonton.

**Opt for cultured yogurt.** Yogurt with live cultures may also help boost the immune system. In one study, after 68 people ate 2 cups of live-culture yogurt daily for three months, they produced more gamma interferon—a substance produced by disease-fighting white blood cells—than people who ate heat-treated yogurt with no active culture, reports the *International Journal of Immunotherapy*. Results persisted two months after people quit eating the yogurt, says George Halpern, M.D., adjunct professor of medicine in the department of internal medicine at the University of California, Davis. He thinks the bacteria in yogurt stimulate parts of the immune system in the intestinal tract.

---

**ANTI-AGING CHECKUP**
# GAUGING YOUR IMMUNITY

There are numerous tests to discover specific strengths and weaknesses of the immune system, but the simplest and most inexpensive is the complete blood count (CBC). This test reveals the number of white blood cells you have, which alerts your doctor to any imbalances in your immune system.

Other tests can measure the effectiveness of your T-cells—a type of white blood cell that's important in the immune system—and detect the presence of individual immune cells and immune chemicals. Doctors can also test for deficiencies of specific nutrients.

# 21

# KNEE PROBLEMS

A KO for Knee Pain

**Anyone**—whether professional athlete, neighborhood jogger, mall walker or department-store salesperson—is vulnerable to some kind of knee problem.

Your knees take a pounding just getting you through an ordinary day. Studies show that your knees absorb the equivalent of three to six times your body weight with every step you take. That means a 150-pound man transfers 900 pounds of weight to his knees with every step. Run or jump, and the impact is even greater.

The problem is that the knees aren't built to withstand many of the pressures put on them. "For many of the demands we place on our knees, we need a joint that's rugged, like the hip, which is a ball-and-socket design with inherent stability," writes James M. Fox, M.D., in *Save Your Knees*. "Instead, we get two giant bones propped on top of another, held together with the anatomical equivalent of rubber bands."

Everything in the knee joint—the kneecap, the rubber-band-like ligaments and the menisci pads that provide cushioning between the bones—is at risk of injury. Sometimes all three are damaged in a single incident. Obviously, the prudent course for every health-conscious person is a knee-strengthening program specially geared to prevent common injuries and speed the healing of any existing problem.

### PROTECT THE CUSHIONING PADS

"Most knee injuries fall into one of two categories: overuse or traumatic," says Lyle Micheli, M.D., associate professor of orthopedic medicine and director of the sports medicine division at Harvard Medical School. Here's how you can help reduce the risk of injury.

**Follow the "10 percent" rule.** "Many people suffer an injury as a result of a training error. They train too hard or go too fast," explains Dr. Micheli. He recommends this standard rule: Never increase the amount you run, walk, swim or weight-lift more than 10 percent each week. So if you're walking 10 miles this week, you shouldn't do more than 11 miles next week.

Overdoing it can cause runner's knee, the most common overuse knee injury. It surfaces as either a dull ache or sharp pain in the kneecap, says Dr. Micheli. The cause is repeated impact from the femur (thighbone) and tibia (shinbone) on parts of the menisci, which makes these pads soften and causes pain in the kneecap.

**Build up your muscles.** Flabby quadriceps and loose hamstring muscles (located in the front and back of the thigh, respectively) both contribute to runner's knee and to most other knee problems. "Weak muscles can't provide the support bones and joints require," says Harris H. McIlwain, M.D., a rheumatologist and joint expert practicing in Tampa. "Consequently, the primary impact of each step is transferred to the bones and cartilage, instead of being supported by the muscles."

**Remember your hamstrings.** Many of those who work out regularly neglect the hamstring muscles, which should be about 60 percent as strong as the quadriceps, according to Spanky Stevens, head trainer at the University of Texas at Tyler. The resulting imbalance between these muscles leads to many knee injuries.

Weight machines make it easy to avoid this imbalance: Leg extension exercises, where you're sitting and raise a weight with your legs, strengthen the quads; leg curls, where you lie on your stomach and pull a weight toward your bottom with your knees, strengthen the hamstrings. You should do both exercises and ensure that the weight you lift with your hamstrings is around 60 percent of what you lift with your quads. For example, if you lift 50 pounds with your quads, you should be able to curl 30 pounds with your hamstrings. If you can't, hold back on developing the quads until your hamstrings are stronger.

**Do some slow, easy stretches.** While lack of fitness certainly opens the knees to increased vulnerability, simple tightness in the joints is also a danger. A lack of flexibility in the tendons and ligaments paves the way to disabling injury of the knees in even the most ordinary activities, says Dr. Micheli.

**Eat less, exercise more.** Osteoarthritis, caused by wear and tear of the joints, often occurs in the knee, either from overuse or from a past injury. Being overweight places an increased burden on the knees and helps wear out cartilage prematurely. Once the surface of the cartilage is worn away, the bones lack protection and grind against each other. The friction can deform bone and cause hardened growths, called spurs, on the bone.

Dr. McIlwain says that if he could prescribe one treatment for arthritis, he'd recommend exercise. "Exercise is one of the most underused treatments available today and one of the most important. By maintaining an exercise program, you make the muscles in the joints flexible, limber and strong, which supports the joints and reduces the pain," he says. (See chapter 3.)

## How to Rehab Bad Knees

Orthopedists recommend that you see an orthopedic specialist or family doctor immediately after incurring a knee injury. Your doctor may recommend some of the following treatments.

**Keep moving.** "I like to keep people going," said Edward J. Resnick, M.D., an orthopedic surgeon at Temple University Hospital in Philadelphia. "As long as the program is kept within certain limits and you avoid overuse, moderate exercise can actually help mitigate the possibility of osteoarthritis, which can easily set in once an injury has occurred. Also, bone, cartilage, tendons and muscles are kept in better condition when they are used and tend to weaken from disuse."

**Massage your knee back to health.** Gently massaging the muscles of the injured knee will speed recovery, writes Dr. Fox in *Save Your Knees*. The massage acts as a "mechanical cleanser," helping the body rid itself of toxins and wastes, improves the blood flow to the tissues and helps lessen inflammation.

**Stretch the hamstrings and calves.** Dr. Resnick suggests this exercise: Stand facing a wall, with both feet together about 18 inches from the wall. Lean forward, using your hands for support, while keeping *both* heels on the floor and knees straight. Adjust your position so that you feel the tug on the muscles of your calves and the back of your thighs.

To modify this exercise, place one foot a little farther back and lean forward while you bend the knee nearest to the wall. This will stretch the hamstring and calf muscles of the leg farthest from the wall. Remember to keep your heel on the ground. Reverse the leg positions to stretch the other leg.

**Do isometrics for knees.** For those just starting a knee-strengthening program or those who have already suffered an injury, Dr. Fox recommends the following isometric exercise. First, sit on the floor, against a wall, with your legs straight out. For support, place a pillow between the small of your back and the wall.

Begin by tightening the muscles of one leg. Tighten those muscles even further. Now, without using your hands, raise your leg so your heel is 4 inches off the floor. Hold it there a few seconds or more, while maintaining the tension in your leg. Lower your leg without releasing the tension. Now try to tighten the leg muscles even more. Finally, relax the leg. Repeat the exercise using your other leg. Your goal is to do 2 sets of 10 repetitions.

**Work out in water.** Among the best rehabilitation exercises are those performed in water because water makes the body weigh less. A wet workout can strengthen leg muscles and improve flexibility without placing pressure directly on the knee.

### Step Up the Effort

As your knee strength improves, you can begin more demanding exercises, such as stair climbing and walking up hills. Here are tips to help you strengthen your knees.

**Lift weights with your ankles.** Sit on the edge of a chair or table, with your legs hanging freely. Wearing ankle weights up to 10 pounds, raise one leg. If you have no pain, extend it straight out; if you do have pain, raise it to only two-thirds of its full extension. Hold it there for 6 seconds, and then rest. Repeat with the other leg. Work your way up to 10 repetitions.

**Do leg raises.** Lie on the floor on your back, legs straight out. Bend one leg at the knee, keeping your foot on the floor. Keep the other leg straight. Raise the straight leg from the hip so your foot is no more than 6 to 8 inches off the floor, and hold for 6 seconds. Rest 6 seconds and repeat. Do 10 repetitions for each leg.

As you gain strength, you can add ankle weights of up to 5 pounds. To make the workout even tougher, hold up your leg without shaking for 10 seconds.

**Vary direction.** Walking or running backward strengthens the hamstrings, according to Stevens. And regardless of which direction you're running, if you're doing it on a track, reverse your direction every other lap. Tracks tend to have a slope from side to bank, which puts more stress on one knee than the other. By reversing the direction, you give both legs equal treatment.

**Protect your feet.** Buy shoes that fit and provide lots of support to save wear and tear on your knees. (See chapter 16.) Also, if you run, stick to soft surfaces, such as earth, grass, wood chips or a track, especially after suffering an injury.

**Wear a seat belt.** Buckling up snugly every time you get in a car is not only an excellent safety maneuver but will also protect against "dashboard knee," an injury that frequently occurs in car accidents when front-seat passengers are thrown forward into the dashboard.

**Avoid knee braces.** Braces can be helpful to protect the knee after an injury, but regularly wearing them for athletic endeavors such as softball or volleyball can cause more trouble than they prevent. What you think is providing extra sup-

ort can actually weaken the muscles of that leg, says Dr.
Resnick, making an injury more likely. Unless you're injured
or your doctor has recommended a brace, leave it at home.

## ANTI-AGING CHECKUP
# DO *YOU* HAVE KNEE PROBLEMS?

While wearing shorts, look in a mirror to check your legs'
alignment. If you have knock-knee, bowlegs or turned-out tib-
ias, you know you are at special risk for encountering knee
problems. Your best protective measure is regular exercise
designed to make your legs stronger and more flexible.

If you suspect osteoarthritis of the knee, answer these questions Yes or No.

____ Do you have persistent pain and swelling in the knees,
especially upon waking or at night?
____ Do you feel pain and stiffness when you flex the knee?
____ Are you unable to move the knee normally?

### INTERPRETING YOUR ANSWERS

If you have these symptoms, see a doctor experienced in de-
tecting and treating knee problems; you could stave off irre-
versible damage.

# 22

# LEG CRAMPS

Muscles That Go "Boing" in the Night

**Most** of us are familiar with the feeling. You're sleeping peacefully, when suddenly you're awakened by a stabbing pain in your calf or foot.

Medical books call these painful involuntary skeletal muscle contractions, but most of us know them as charley horses or simply cramps. Leg cramps affect millions of Americans and are not only a painful nuisance, they can destroy your chances of a good night's sleep. They're the fourth leading cause of insomnia, according to the journal *Clinical Pharmacy*.

Cramps are a mysterious phenomenon, striking trained athletes as well as older people who might overdo physical activity on a weekend. Cramps occur while a person is resting, often at night, and affect the calf and foot muscles. Each cramp lasts only a few seconds but can interrupt sleep nightly for a few days or weeks, then mysteriously disappear. In some unlucky souls, night cramps occur for months or even years. The affliction is particularly prevalent in people past middle age and in pregnant women.

Most leg cramps fall into one of two categories: ordinary cramps, referred to as nocturnal cramps because they often occur at night; or cramps caused by arteries in the legs being clogged by cholesterol plaque. Let's first take a look at ordinary leg cramps and what you can do about them.

## WHY THE CRAMP STRIKES

Ordinary cramps usually occur in the first few hours of sleep. For unknown reasons, your leg or foot muscles seize up.

But scientists have some theories as to why these cramps occur. Cramps are prolonged muscle contractions, brought on by commands within the nervous system. Normally, the brain sends a signal via the nervous system to a specific set of muscles, ordering those muscles to perform a certain task. Once the job is done, the brain sends another signal telling the muscle to relax.

But a cramped muscle is already contracted, and instead of being told to relax, it is ordered by nerve cells to continue to contract, which sends the muscle into a painful spasm. This is why your first impulse—to stretch the affected muscle—usually brings relief.

Scientists believe these prolonged contractions are a result of imbalances in the body's supply of certain minerals, called electrolytes, which make electrical impulses in the nervous system possible. Among the most important of these are calcium, potassium and sodium.

Circumstantial evidence supports this theory. Cramps sometimes occur in athletes who overexercise or sweat profusely, suggesting that the loss of sodium in sweat plays a role in causing some cramps. Also, certain medications that affect electrolyte balance are associated with increased cramping.

## DRUG-FREE STRATEGIES FOR RELIEF

Some people treat leg cramps with a drug called quinine, but it may have side effects, including headaches, unsteady gait, nausea, vision problems, uneven heartbeat, low blood pressure and, in extreme cases, even blindness. It works in only about 50 percent of cases, says Harry Daniell, M.D., clinical professor in the department of family practice at the University of California Medical School at Davis. Instead, try these ways to vanquish cramps.

**Stretch, then relax.** Place both hands on a wall you're facing, with one foot about 2 feet from the wall, the other about 3 feet from the wall. Lean forward as you bend the knee of the leg closest to the wall. Keep the other leg straight, with the heel touching the floor. This will stretch the calf and heel muscles of that leg. Hold the position for 10 seconds, and relax for 5. Repeat with the opposite leg. Repeat 2 or 3 times for each leg. Try doing 5 to 10 of these stretches just before bed.

**Take a walk.** One of the best ways to gently stretch your leg muscles is walking. Don't overdo it; start out slowly.

**Try a massage.** Massage the affected muscle with a warming salve such as Ben-Gay.

**Change your position.** Don't sleep on your stomach. This puts your calf muscles into a shortened position, where they're more likely to cramp.

**Drink up.** Drink six to eight glasses of fluid every day. Dehydration predisposes you to cramps.

**Be prepared.** Keep a towel or scarf at your bedside. If you get a severe cramp during the night, put the cloth under the front of your foot and pull up your toes until the cramp is gone.

**Consider supplements.** Although there's no definitive scientific proof, you might consider supplements of certain nutrients—1,500 milligrams of calcium and 400 international units of vitamin E daily—says Dr. Daniell. "Again, no one knows why these nutrients may work, but they often do. Since people need both in their diets, and since they are safe in these quantities, I sometimes suggest people take them," he says.

**Pump up your intake of certain nutrients.** Dr. Daniell recommends that people try to eat more foods that contain calcium, magnesium and potassium to cut leg cramps. (Sodium is also important, but unless you eat no processed foods and don't use salt, you get plenty in your diet.)

**Raise your feet.** Prop your feet higher than your head when in bed. You can do this either by sleeping with your legs on a pillow or pillows or by putting books or a board under the end of your bed.

**Pull on some support.** Wear calf-high support hose or support socks.

## A DIFFERENT KIND OF CRAMP

Now let's take a look at cramps caused by cholesterol plaque in the legs, called claudication. Claudication—named for the Roman emperor Claudius, who was lame—occurs after you've walked a certain distance. As mentioned in the chapter on circulation, the cause is atherosclerosis, or cholesterol plaque inside the arteries of the legs.

Because the arteries carrying oxygen-rich blood are blocked with plaque, the muscles are deprived of the oxygen they need to keep you walking. Consequently, the muscles in your legs or buttocks cramp, a protest you can't ignore. The pain disappears once you've rested for a while, but it resumes after you walk a short distance, even a few hundred feet. Because the pain comes and goes, this is also called intermittent claudication.

What causes the plaque? Although the pain occurs during walking, a lack of exercise—in addition to smoking and a high-fat, high-cholesterol diet—contributes to causing the problem in the first place. By changing your habits, you may help your claudication problem and lower your risk for heart disease or stroke as well. (See chapter 8 for ways to improve your diet and chapter 23 for smoking-cessation tips.)

Suffering from claudication doesn't mean you have to stay home in your armchair. The road back to improved function is exercise, says Eugene Strandness, Jr., M.D., professor of surgery at the University of Washington School of Medicine in Seattle. "Walking improves endurance and increases the distance you can go," he says. Walking will help your muscles utilize oxygen and nutrients more efficiently—and it may even cause more blood vessels to grow in your legs, increasing the amount of blood and oxygen flowing to your muscles. Dr. Strandness recommends the following walking program.

**First, cut your distance.** If you can walk only a block with pain, just walk three-fourths of a block and rest. Then walk another three-fourths of a block and rest again. Do that same routine four times. The reason you walk only three-quarters of your maximum is that you want to stop short of the level at which your muscles are deprived of oxygen and go into a cramp. Repeat the whole process twice a day for one week.

**ANTI-AGING CHECKUP**
# DON'T IGNORE LEG CRAMPS

Frequent leg cramps may indicate a circulatory problem called claudication that should be treated by a doctor. To find out if your cramps are more than just cramps, answer these questions Yes or No.

_____ Do your feet feel cold to the touch?

_____ Has the hair below your knees stopped growing?

_____ Does the skin over your shins appear thin, smooth and shiny?

_____ When you press the fleshy part of your big toe firmly, does the skin turn white and then take a long time to return to pink?

_____ When your feet are dangling, are they dusky red in color? And if you immediately elevate them, do they look very pale:

## INTERPRETING YOUR ANSWERS

If the answer to any of these questions is Yes, consult your doctor.

**Find your new maximum.** After a week, retest yourself by walking until you experience pain. This is your new maximum walking distance, which may now be a little more than a block.

**Keep extending yourself.** For the following week, do the same exercise twice a day, but walk three-fourths of your new maximum distance. Each week, retest yourself and keep extending your three-fourths maximum distance. You will see rapid improvements in the distance you can walk without pain.

# 23

# LUNGS

## How to Breathe Easy

**First,** the not-so-good news: No matter how much you exercise or avoid cigarettes and passive smoking, odds are you're still going to lose some lung capacity as you age.

The reasons are simple. As we age, "the elastic properties of the lungs change," says John Sharp, M.D., professor of medicine, physiology and biophysics at the University of Southern Florida in Tampa. "The lungs don't snap back as well. As we grow older, they become like an overstretched rubber band."

The condition of the muscles in our chest also affects our breathing. The ability of the muscles to expand and contract influences how much oxygen we can take in. And that's where the good news comes in. While the strength of these muscles also tends to lessen with age, their relative fitness can be preserved with exercise and maintenance of overall health.

In fact, there's a lot you can do to preserve your lung capacity. Even some folks with certain types of lung disease, such as emphysema, can lesson the symptoms of illness and improve lung function.

### TAKE SLOW, DEEP BREATHS

Many people breathe rapidly and shallowly, a condition called hyperventilation syndrome (HVS). These people get less oxygen than others who breathe more slowly and deeply. Because oxygen is used to produce energy, people with HVS are often fatigued. Shallow breathing has been linked to a variety of other conditions, including anxiety, poor circulation, kidney disease, anemia, diabetes and hypertension. Here are four ways to combat this problem.

**Take a hike.** Or a bike ride, a jog or a swim. One way to train yourself to breathe better is to get regular aerobic exercise, which forces you to inhale and exhale deeply and strengthens chest muscles.

**Train for best-in-breathing rewards.** You can also practice emptying and filling your lungs, exhaling most of the retained carbon dioxide to make more room for oxygen. Stand up straight, and slowly exhale until all your breath is gone. Then slowly breathe in until your chest is expanded as far as it will go. Do this a few times a day.

**"Watch" yourself breathe.** While sitting or standing, put one hand on your chest and the other on your abdomen. Watch your hands as you breathe; both should rise and fall simultaneously. If only the hand on your chest rises—or if it rises higher than the hand on your stomach—you may be taking those undesirable rapid, shallow breaths and hyperventilating.

**Let your nose do the breathing.** One of the causes of short, shallow breaths is breathing through the mouth, says Robert Fried, Ph.D., of the Institute for Rational Emotive Therapy in New York and author of *The Breath Connection* and *The Hyperventilation Syndrome*. You can cure yourself of such breathing by taking care to breathe only through your nose.

## BREAK THE HABIT THAT'S LETHAL TO LUNGS

Smoking actually breaks down tissues within the lungs and causes the destruction of the tiny air sacs (alveoli) in the lungs, says Dr. Sharp. Smoking is the leading cause of emphysema, an illness that destroys the alveoli. Emphysema also causes the lungs to lose elasticity, resulting in diminished oxygen intake.

Needless to say, smoking not only stands in the way of staying young, it prevents you from staying *alive*. Lung cancer causes more than 350,000 deaths yearly—most due to smoking. More than nine out of ten cases of lung cancers are fatal because they generally go undetected until they reach an advanced stage. With each puff, *hundreds* of cancer-causing chemicals in cigarette smoke are absorbed into the blood-stream.

Ready to kick the habit? Experts recommend these ways to help you quit.

**Set a target date.** Post "quit smoking" reminders in prominent places at home and office as a frequent reminder of your intention. Then, on the appointed day, toss the cigarettes.

---

**ANTI-AGING CHECKUP**
# TAKE THE BALLOON TEST

According to British researchers, blowing up a small balloon 40 times a day for eight weeks will not only dramatically improve your lung capacity but also serve as a graphic self-test for the condition of your lungs and provide a well-defined yardstick for your progress.

The researchers compared 28 people with respiratory conditions. Thirteen of them blew up a small balloon to a diameter of 20 centimeters (about 8 inches), 40 times a day. At both the start and conclusion of the study, walking tests were administered on both groups. After eight weeks, the researchers found that the 13 who blew up balloons fared better on the walking test for speed and endurance, experienced less breathlessness and had higher scores for well-being than the other 15 study participants.

If you try this exercise, try your own before-and-after walking test (walk for a specific time, and see how far you go and how you feel), and watch the strength of your lungs improve.

---

**Take up a sport.** Adopt an exercise program, especially if you rely on smoking to give you a lift. The high you get from natural "feel good" chemicals released by exercise will replace the stimulating lift you may be accustomed to getting from nicotine.

**Examine your motives.** Each time you feel the impulse to light up, ask yourself if you really want a cigarette. You'll be surprised at how many times the answer is no. Often you're smoking merely out of habit.

**Consider nicotine spray.** Ask your doctor about the self-administered nicotine nasal spray, which reduces the craving for a cigarette. According to a study published in the British medical journal *Lancet,* it was twice as effective at helping people give up cigarettes as a spray without nicotine. "Nasal nicotine spray combined with supportive group treatment is an effective aid to smoking cessation," concluded the researchers.

**Try nicotine gum.** If you're truly addicted to smoking, nicotine gum may help you quit. Some studies show that half the people who use the gum are able to stop smoking. (Acid-rich food or drink, however, will neutralize the nicotine in the gum before it is absorbed into your bloodstream. So avoid consuming colas, milk, beer, coffee, chicken soup, lemon-lime soda and fruit juices for at least 30 minutes before chewing the gum.)

**Put on a nicotine patch.** Ask your doctor about a nicotine patch. When used in conjunction with other stop-smoking measures, this can be an effective aid for people who find it tough to quit. Follow instructions carefully to minimize adverse effects. Continuing to smoke while wearing the patch can leave you feeling *very* sick.

**Let your fingers do the walking.** Smoking-cessation programs often include counseling, relaxation training, hypnosis or some other form of behavioral therapy. To explore the range of programs that exist in your area, call your local chapter of the American Cancer Society or the American Lung Association.

**Go cold turkey.** Eighty-five percent of former smokers preferred to stop completely, with no aids. Many people respond best to a tough challenge. Dare yourself to quit—and *do* it.

# 24

# MENOPAUSE

### Ease Your Way
### through the Change of Life

**Menopause** is as natural as birth, puberty and adulthood, but misconceptions still exist about a woman's "change of life" and the symptoms that usually accompany it. Many women regard menopause as a medical condition or something to be suffered through rather than a natural process whose challenges can be navigated safely and gracefully.

Menopause marks the time when a woman's ovaries stop producing eggs and significantly decrease their production of estrogen, the female hormone, and menstruation stops. Most women reach menopause around age 50 or 51. About one out of ten women reaches menopause early (before age 38), and some don't start until their late 50s, according to Susan Perry and Katharine O'Hanlan, M.D., authors of *Natural Menopause: The Complete Guide to a Woman's Most Misunderstood Passage*. The following factors can speed up or slow down menopause.

**Smoking.** Cigarette smoking decreases the ovaries' production of estrogen and is associated with earlier menopause.

**Weight.** As a group, women whose weight exceeds about 130 pounds tend to experience menopause later than women who weigh less, possibly because fat cells produce estrogen.

**Twin births.** Giving birth to twins is associated with experiencing menopause about a year earlier than other mothers, though no one is really sure why.

Officially, menopause is the 12-month time span after your

last period; after this, you're through menopause. It's the two or more years prior to actual menopause, however, called peri-menopause, when many physical changes take place. Symptoms include irregular and heavy menstrual periods, hot flashes, night sweats, vaginal dryness and thinning of the walls of the vagina. However, these problems can be managed and reduced.

### Learn How to Cope with Heavy Periods

While both heavy bleeding and irregular periods are normal during menopause, some women panic at this. Here are some ways Dr. O'Hanlan recommends to help deal with heavy flow.

**Cut back on alcohol.** Heavy drinking prevents blood from clotting efficiently and can contribute to increased bleeding.

**Skip the aspirin.** Avoid aspirin, which also increases blood flow and reduces the blood's ability to clot. Instead, use aceta-minophen for pain.

**Stay out of hot water.** Avoid hot showers, hot baths, and hot compresses because heat increases blood flow.

**Get regular checkups.** Bleeding can be a sign of health issues that are unrelated to menopause. Your doctor should be consulted to rule out other possible causes, such as cancer of the cervix, uterus or ovaries, liver problems or disorders of the blood-clotting system.

**Check out your iron levels.** Heavy periods can reduce the iron content of the blood and may result in fatigue, depression or anemia. You can get more of this mineral by eating red meat, clams or dark leafy greens and by using iron pots, which leach iron into food during cooking (particularly if an acidic food such as tomatoes is cooked in them). Don't take iron supplements unless a blood test has demonstrated that your stores are low, however.

### Control Your Inner Thermostat

Though scientists are not entirely sure why hot flashes occur, they believe that the hypothalamus, the master gland in the brain, mistakenly signals the body to kick its natural cooling mechanisms into gear. The body sets in motion an array of cooling responses, including increases in heart rate, circulation and perspiration. When this happens, your skin temperature heats up a full eight degrees, while your internal temperature drops. The result? That out-of-the-blue heat spell known as a hot flash.

Though they can be frightening and uncomfortable, these hot flashes are perfectly harmless. (When not related to menopause, hot flashes can be a sign of illness and should be reported to your doctor.) Here are some tips to alleviate your discomfort.

**Wear cotton for comfort.** Cotton garments let your skin breathe better than synthetics do and allow the body to better regulate its temperature.

**Quit smoking.** Cigarette smoking constricts blood vessels, which can prolong and intensify hot flashes.

**Steer clear of caffeine.** Some women report that foods and drinks containing caffeine, such as chocolate, coffee, teas and colas, may set off a hot flash.

**Track your flashes.** Keeping a record of when and under what conditions you experience hot flashes may help you understand what triggers them and help you manage them. Note how long the spell lasts, how intense it is and what circumstances and feelings preceded it. Certain foods may affect you, for instance. Many women report that sugar and alcohol can trigger hot flashes.

**Stay out of the heat.** Avoid areas of extreme heat, such as saunas, Jacuzzis and very hot baths.

**Take a deep breath.** Slow, deep breathing can dramatically reduce the intensity and frequency of hot flashes, says Robert R. Freedman, Ph.D., professor of psychiatry at the Lafayette Clinic and Wayne State University School of Medicine in Detroit. A group of 33 women experiencing frequent hot flashes practiced either slow, deep breathing, muscle relaxation or biofeedback. The latter two had no effect, while deep breathing resulted in half as many flashes.

The technique is simple and easy: Just cut your breathing rate in half. Instead of taking 14 to 16 breaths per minute, take 6 to 8. "The key is to breathe from your belly instead of your chest," says Dr. Freedman. "That creates a deeper, more relaxing breath." Practice twice a day until it comes naturally, and when you feel a hot flash coming on—during stressful moments or in a hot room—take slow, deep breaths.

## GUARD YOUR BONES

One serious concern related to menopause is bone health and the prevention of osteoporosis, brittle bones that occur primarily after menopause.

How can you protect your bones? "You need good nutrition, including calcium, healthy hormone levels and several kinds of exercise," says Gail Dalsky, Ph.D., director of the exercise research lab at the University of Connecticut Health Center's Osteoporosis Center.

**Exercise is crucial.** "The evidence that exercise is beneficial to bone is overwhelming," says Sydney Lou Bonnick, M.D., director of osteoporosis services at the Cooper Clinic in Dallas. "You can maintain or even increase your bone mass through appropriate exercises."

Weight-bearing endurance exercise is effective, including walking, dancing, jogging, aerobic dance or vigorous tennis. Resistance training may be even more powerful.

**Work out *and* increase your calcium intake.** Scientists have found that the combination of regular exercise and a calcium-rich diet is the best formula for preventing bone loss and increasing bone density. Most women should get 1,000 milligrams of calcium per day; women past menopause who are not on hormone replacement therapy should get 1,500 milligrams daily.

Good sources of calcium include skim-milk products, collard greens, kale, broccoli, tofu, sardines (if you eat the bones), beans, figs and almonds. If you take a supplement, do not exceed 2,500 milligrams because excess calcium may cause constipation or possibly kidney stones.

**Remember your D.** To help your body absorb and use calcium, you must have vitamin D. Your skin manufactures this vitamin when exposed to the sun's ultraviolet rays. Exposing your face, arms and hands to the sun (without sunscreen) for five to ten minutes a day, three times a week, will provide an adequate dose. Many experts recommend that you enjoy the sunlight in the morning or late afternoon to avoid the adverse effects of too many ultraviolet rays. You can also get your quota from fortified milk or in a multivitamin with 200 to 400 international units of vitamin D.

### WEIGH THE PROS AND CONS OF HRT

It's the dramatic drop in estrogen that occurs during menopause that causes most of the symptoms. Consequently, hormone replacement therapy (HRT), which provides estrogen and progesterone in the form of progestin, will significantly reduce or completely eliminate many adverse effects of menopause. HRT can be administered as tablets, a gel that's applied daily or a patch worn on the skin for 72 hours, twice a week.

---

## KEEPING SEXUALLY ACTIVE

Menopause doesn't have to negatively impact your sex life, but because one of the natural consequences of menopause is vaginal dryness, you may want to make some changes in how you approach intercourse.

Using a sterile, water-soluble jelly (such as K-Y Jelly or Astro-Glide) can relieve vaginal dryness. These products can be applied both externally and internally, before or during sex.

Also, the longer the foreplay before intercourse, the more time the body has to produce its own lubricants. Women in their 50s can still produce natural lubrication, according to research by experts; they just need a little more time than women in their 20s.

---

HRT has also been shown to reduce bone loss and protect against heart disease and stroke. On the down side, there is an increased incidence of breast cancer among women who take HRT; also, possible side effects include weight gain, depression and migraine headaches.

Not all menopause women need HRT. Ovaries don't completely stop making estrogen during menopause, and the adrenal glands, which sit on top of the kidneys, partially compensate by making androstenedione, a hormone the body converts into estrogen. Together, the ovaries and adrenals may produce enough estrogen to maintain healthy bones without HRT, as long as diet and exercise prescriptions are followed.

HRT can be recommended only after a woman's personal and family medical histories are carefully considered. Factors to be taken into account include a personal or family history of breast or uterine cancer, heart disease, stroke or high blood pressure or cigarette smoking. Discuss these issues with your doctor before taking HRT.

---

### ANTI-AGING CHECKUP
## ARE YOU GOING THROUGH THE CHANGE?

Because not all women experience menopause at the same age, it is sometimes difficult to know with certainty if you are experiencing its early symptoms. Answer the following Yes or No to help you determine whether or not you are undergoing the early stages. Do you experience:

\_\_\_\_ Heavy or prolonged menstrual flows?

\_\_\_\_ Periods that are longer than usual and fewer than 21 days apart? (When figuring the number of days between periods, you should count from the first day of your previous period to the first day of your current period.)

\_\_\_\_ Bleeding or spotting between periods?

\_\_\_\_ Unusual cramping during menstruation?

\_\_\_\_ Bleeding that occurs again after you have gone 12 months without a period? (This can be a sign of a tumor.)

### INTERPRETING YOUR ANSWERS

If you experience any of these symptoms, experts say, see your gynecologist, especially if you are in your late 30s or early 50s.

# 25

# NUTRITION

Top Stay-Young Diet Strategies

**If** Ponce de León were around today, he could end his search for the Fountain of Youth in just about any grocery store.

Scientific evidence is mounting that the right foods offer many of the very benefits that the Spanish explorer searched for in vain, including protection against heart disease, cancer, arthritis, osteoporosis, cataracts and other illnesses *assumed* to accompany aging. Scientists now believe that an anti-aging diet can keep us younger, stronger and healthier longer.

"In many cases, nutrition is a new form of medicine," says William Pryor, Ph.D., professor of chemistry and biochemistry and director of the Biodynamics Institute at Louisiana State University in Baton Rouge. "Now we're finding that the effects of certain nutrients are quite potent and, in many cases, will reduce the incidence of disease by about 50 percent."

How can nutrition help? The same process that causes iron to rust—oxidation—occurs in our bodies, resulting in unstable molecules called free radicals. When there are too many free radicals, they can attack and break down body cells. More and more scientists are beginning to believe that free radicals are at least partly responsible for many health problems previously blamed on other factors (like fate).

Certain nutrients called antioxidants, however, can latch on to the free radicals and render them harmless. Conversely, some foods, such as saturated fat, speed up the production of free radicals.

In addition, researchers are discovering that certain foods

and herbs contain other disease-fighting properties that fight cancer, heart disease and other major illnesses.

## MEET A TRIO OF POWERFUL NUTRIENTS

Vitamins C, E and beta-carotene (a nutrient found in vegetables that converts to vitamin A in the body) are among a group of powerful antioxidants that prevent the formation of free radicals and prevent or slow many illnesses. Antioxidants have been shown to prevent atherosclerosis—the underlying cause of heart disease—and boost the immune system in a variety of ways. Here's the lowdown.

**Give your immune system a boost.** Antioxidants slow aging and protect against disease by boosting the immune system. "Generally, immunity declines somewhat as we get older, making us more susceptible to bacterial and viral infections as well as certain diseases most common among the elderly, like cancer, arthritis and heart disease," explains Jeffrey Blumberg, Ph.D., associate director of the U.S. Department of Agriculture's Human Nutrition Research Center on Aging at Tufts University in Boston.

Studies have shown that certain nutrients, especially the powerful trio mentioned above, may slow or prevent the decline in immunity. "Our most striking work in this area was with vitamin E supplements in older people," says Dr. Blumberg. "We found that high doses markedly improved certain tests of immune function."

**Every little bit helps.** Even a single daily serving of fruits or vegetables rich in beta-carotene may reduce your risk of heart attack and stroke, according to the Nurses' Health Study, which involved 87,245 women. "We found a 22 percent reduction in the risk of heart attack and a 40 percent reduction in stroke for those women with high intakes of fruits and vegetables rich in beta-carotene, compared with those with low intakes," says JoAnn E. Manson, M.D., one of the doctors involved in the heart section of the study, which was done for Brigham and Women's Hospital and Harvard Medical School.

**C can benefit your heart.** Research suggests that vitamin C boosts HDL cholesterol, the "good" cholesterol that prevents atherosclerotic plaques from forming in your arteries, and stops LDL cholesterol, the kind that creates blockages in the arteries and leads to heart attack and stroke. A study published in the *Journal of the American College of Nutrition* involving 1,372 people (850 were over age 60) showed that a higher intake of vitamin C was linked with higher levels of HDL, lower LDL and lower blood pressure. Good C sources include broccoli, brussels sprouts, cauliflower, green peppers, strawberries and orange juice.

**Vitamin E helps keep hearts healthy.** Low blood levels of vitamin E are associated with more than twice the risk of angina (chest pains usually caused by reduced blood flow to the heart muscle) and greater incidence of coronary heart disease, states a report in the British medical journal *Lancet.* One theory is that vitamin E helps keep blood from clotting too easily, which allows it to flow through narrowed coronary arteries.

In a Harvard Medical School study of nearly 40,000 men, those with the lowest risk of heart disease had vitamin E intakes of 60 to 100 international units (I.U.) per day. And in the women studied in the Nurses' Health Study, those who took daily supplements of 100 I.U. had a 36 percent lower risk of heart attack than those who didn't take supplements.

You can get vitamin E from sunflower seeds, sweet potatoes, vegetable oils, whole grains, kale and spinach.

## Cut Cancer Risks

Research has consistently shown that diet plays a major role in both the cause and prevention of cancer, especially common cancers of the breast, colon and prostate. Diets that are rich in fat and low in fiber, antioxidants and certain minerals *raise* your risk of cancer.

Swedish scientists who for 15 years compared the eating habits of 41 people with colorectal cancer with a group of cancer-free people concluded that those who ate diets richer in fiber, calcium and phosphorus were less likely to get cancer. Certain substances in fruits and vegetables, especially fiber and antioxidants, apparently also protect against breast cancer. When researchers at the State University of New York at Buffalo compared the eating habits of 310 women with breast cancer with 316 cancer-free women, they found that the women without cancer ate significantly more vegetables, fruits and fiber.

Here are some ways to lower your cancer risks.

**Put beans on the menu.** Hispanic women, who have lower rates of breast cancer than Caucasian women, also eat twice as many beans as Caucasians, say scientists at the American Health Foundation in New York. Beans contain high amounts of estrogen-blocking substances called phyto-estrogens, which may protect against cancer.

**Cook with garlic.** Studies have found lower rates of stomach and colorectal cancers among those who eat lots of garlic. Scientists speculate that garlic may block the tumor-producing effects of a certain prostaglandin. (Prostaglandins are essential fatty acids, but this particular one can "go bad" and encourage tumor growth.)

Research suggests that the sulfur compounds in garlic can inhibit prostaglandin metabolism, says Herbert Pierson, Ph.D., formerly with the National Cancer Institute in Bethesda, Maryland, and now with Preventive Nutrition Consultants in Rockville. "They may also enhance parts of our immune system and intercept carcinogens when they're activated in our body, preventing them from damaging our cells," says Dr. Pierson.

Both raw and cooked garlic have health-enhancing properties. Scientists recommend using garlic both ways—eating it raw and sautéed in, say, vegetables or spaghetti sauce.

**Load up on cruciferous veggies.** These include broccoli, cabbage, kale, brussels sprouts and collard and mustard greens. These vegetables contain a group of compounds, called indoles, that may prevent tumor-causing estrogen from targeting the breast. In animal studies, they have been shown to switch on enzymes that prevent exposure to carcinogens. Cruciferous vegetables are also rich sources of another cancer-fighter called sulforanphane, which may help cleanse tissues and blood and promote production of enzymes that help prevent cancer.

**Fight cancer with phytochemicals.** Phytochemicals are substances found in plants that may protect them against stresses, climate and infection, and researchers believe these substances may help people as well. Foods rich in phytochemicals are soybeans, carrots, parsnips, celery and parsley. To reduce cancer risks, a combination of these vegetables would probably work best, says Dr. Pierson.

**Sip green tea.** "Many constituents in green tea are capable of blocking cell mutations," Dr. Pierson says. In addition to antioxidants, green tea contains flavonoids, compounds that help prevent cancer in animals.

## GET THE MOST FROM YOUR DIET

So stay-young strategy number one is to build meals around fruits and vegetables, legumes and garlic. Here's what else you can do to ensure that what you eat supplies good nutrition *and* helps you fight disease.

**Try more meatless meals and nonfat dairy products.** Dietary fat produces free radicals in your body, says Dr. Pryor, and is a major cause of premature aging and disease. Not only that, fat can contribute to problems such as clogged arteries and has been linked to heart disease and cancers of the breast, colon and prostate. The average American consumes 80 to 100 grams of fat per day—the equivalent of almost a whole stick of butter!

William Castelli, M.D., director of the Framingham Heart Study, a long-term study gathering health-related data on the adult residents of Framingham, Massachusetts, urges people to read labels and limit fat intake to a maximum of 67 grams per day. Only a third of that (about 22 grams) should be saturated fat. Saturated fats are found in animal foods—red meat, dairy products and eggs—as well as a handful of vegetable foods, such as olives, coconuts and palm-kernel oils. Other experts recommend even *less* fat and saturated fat intake. (See chapters 8 and 19.)

**Fill up with fiber.** Fiber improves intestinal health and lowers blood cholesterol, thus helping to prevent atherosclerosis and coronary heart disease. Fiber can also fend off constipation and can help you lose weight by filling you up. It may cut your risks of breast cancer and colon cancer and, in some cases, can reduce the need for insulin in people with diabetes. (See chapter 11.) Sources of fiber include oatmeal, oat brain, psyllium, legumes such as beans and split peas, vegetables and fruit, whole-grain products and whole grains, including brown rice, bulgur, barley and millet.

---

## THE BEST ANTI-AGING DIET KNOWN

Scientists at the U.S. Department of Agriculture Human Nutrition Research Center at Tufts University in Boston tell us that these four simple rules are good guidelines for an anti-aging diet.

- Get less than 30 percent of your calories from fat.
- Eat foods rich in the antioxidant vitamins C, E and beta-carotene, such as carrots, winter squash, pumpkin, sweet potatoes, spinach, broccoli, cantaloupe and peaches.
- Consume low-fat foods high in calcium, such as low-fat dairy products, collard greens, kale, broccoli and sardines with the bones.
- Increase fiber intake to 20 to 35 grams per day. Excellent high-fiber foods include figs, plums, peaches and legumes.

Some experts also recommend that you take a multi-vitamin-and-mineral supplement to ensure you're getting at least the Recommended Dietary Allowances (RDAs) of all essential nutrients. If you do take a supplement, choose one with no more than 100 percent of the RDAs.

---

**Try some wheat germ.** Wheat germ, a good source of fiber and vitamin E, caused a significant drop in the blood cholesterol and triglyceride (harmful blood fat) levels of 19 people studied by scientists at the National Institute of Health and Medical Research in Marseilles, France. Although these people ate a high-fat diet (40 percent of their calories from fat), cholesterol levels fell an average of 8 percent after four weeks of eating 20 grams of wheat germ a day (about 3 tablespoons). When the wheat germ intake was bumped to 30 grams a day, triglyceride levels fell 11.3 percent.

**Select finned food.** Fish contains omega-3 fatty acids, a type of polyunsaturated fat that may help prevent heart disease. Studies have linked high fish consumption with lower incidences of heart disease and stroke in Greenland Eskimos and Japanese fishermen.

Low-fat fish such as sole, haddock and cod are an excellent protein source, with less cholesterol and fat than lean red meat. A 3-ounce serving of very lean ground beef, for example, has 70 milligrams of cholesterol, 5.4 grams of saturated fat and 13.8 grams of total fat. In contrast, a 3-ounce serving of scallops contains 25 milligrams of cholesterol, 0.07 grams of saturated fat and 0.6 grams of total fat. A big difference!

**Pump in the calcium.** Getting adequate calcium is essential for everyone. It's particularly crucial for women, however, because they are at higher risk of losing bone tissue and developing the brittle-bone condition known as osteoporosis. (See chapter 26.)

Calcium may also help alleviate premenstrual symptoms. In a study at the Human Nutrition Research Center in Grand Forks, North Dakota, researchers assigned ten women to a diet with either 1,300 or 600 milligrams of calcium. Halfway through the 5½-month study, the women switched. The women reported feeling less irritable, anxious and depressed, and seven reported fewer cramps, backaches and headaches when they ate more calcium.

Eating calcium-rich foods may also help people lower mild high blood pressure to normal levels, according to a study at the Oregon Health Sciences University in Portland.

The recommended dietary allowance for calcium is 800 milligrams a day for men and women; pregnant and lactating women should get 1,200 milligrams. Most experts recommend that postmenopausal women consume 1,000 to 1,200 milligrams daily to help ward off osteoporosis. Besides low-fat dairy products, healthy sources of calcium include broccoli, kale, collard greens and sardines or salmon (if you eat the bones).

**Fill up with water.** Water, which is essential to many body processes, has been called the forgotten nutrient. On average, we lose 2 to 3 quarts every day—and usually don't drink enough to replace what we've lost. "The average person is a pint short on water each day, putting stress on the kidneys," says George Blackburn, M.D., Ph.D., chief of the nutrition/metabolism laboratory at New England Deaconess Hospital in Boston and associate professor of medicine at Harvard Medical School. Caffeine-containing beverages such as coffee, tea and some sodas don't help: They're diuretics that promote water loss. To up your fluid intake, drink water rather than another beverage with your meals, or drink a cup of water *before* your other beverage.

**Keep fuel in your tank.** Skipping breakfast is like running your car when it's low on oil and coolant: It may work, but it's tough on the engine. Not only is your body starved for fuel in the morning (whether you *feel* hungry or not), but you're more likely to overeat and grab the wrong foods when you do settle down to a meal. "After five hours without eating, you are subject to ravenous hunger, and you do not care about health goals and good intentions," says Evelyn Tribole, R.D., a nutritionist in private practice in Beverly Hills, California, and author of *Eating on the Run*.

**Cut couch time, not calories.** Losing weight and keeping it off is tricky. Experts recommend that you not try to lose weight simply by cutting back on your eating—you're apt to lose out on too many anti-aging nutrients. Instead, begin exercising as well as reducing your fat and sugar intake.

**Make one small change at a time.** After reading about the near-magical powers of good nutrition, you may feel compelled to make a clean sweep, ridding your diet of processed foods, sugars and fat and hiking your intake of fiber, fruits, vegetables and fish. But trying to change everything at once is likely too big a step, for both your psyche *and* your body. (Rapidly increasing your fiber intake, for example, can cause intestinal distress.) Your best bet is to make one change at a time.

## ANTI-AGING CHECKUP
# AN ANTI-AGING INVENTORY

How does your diet compare with the U.S. Department of Agriculture's (USDA's) guidelines? These guidelines are described by a Food Guide Pyramid, which divides foods into six groups.

At the bottom of the pyramid are the foods that should make up the bulk of your diet: breads, cereals, rice and pasta. Next come fruits, then vegetables, then nonfat or low-fat dairy products. Protein sources such as poultry, fish, legumes, meat, eggs and nuts appear next. At the very tip of the pyramid are fats, oils and sugars—meaning you should keep these foods to a minimum.

To see how your diet stacks up to the USDA recommendations, answer the following questions Yes or No.

_____ Do you eat 6 to 11 servings of grains per day, including bread, cereals, rice and pasta? (One slice of bread equals one serving.)

_____ Do you eat 3 to 5 servings of vegetables daily? (One serving equals 1/2 cup.)

_____ Do you eat 2 to 4 servings of fruit daily? (One serving equals one piece of fruit, 1/2 cup of cut fruit or 3/4 cup of juice.)

_____ Do you eat 2 to 3 servings of milk, yogurt, cheese or other calcium sources daily? (One serving equals 1 cup of milk or 1 cup of yogurt.)

_____ Do you eat 2 to 3 servings of protein foods, such as fish, poultry, meat, dry beans and peas, eggs or nuts, daily? (One serving equals 3 ounces, about the size of a deck of cards.)

_____ Do you keep intake of fats, oils and sugars to a minimum?

## INTERPRETING YOUR ANSWERS

If you answered No to any question, you should probably revise your shopping list before you visit the grocery store and choose different foods when you eat out.

# 26

# OSTEOPOROSIS

### Building Better Bones

**In** our looks-conscious, on-the-go culture, the word thin has all the right connotations—unless you're talking about your bones. Then it can mean one of the most debilitating diseases of modern life: osteoporosis, the gradual thinning and wasting away of bone tissue. What that means, in practical terms, is that the same fall you could take on a sidewalk at age 30 without shattering more than your pride could splinter your wrist at 55 or break your hip at age 85.

Osteoporosis, which affects approximately 25 million Americans, works silently, eroding the mineral content of bones over time. As bones become more porous—the word *osteoporosis* means "porous bone"—they become more vulnerable to fracture.

Each year, osteoporosis is the cause of about 1.5 million fractures; one-third of all U.S. women will suffer a hip fracture. And you don't have to be shredding powder at Jackson Hole, Wyoming, to buckle under. Many of these breaks occur as people perform the most routine tasks—bending down to pick up a newspaper or pushing a shopping cart around the store. Hip fractures are among the most dangerous: Twenty percent result in medical complications that prove fatal. About half of the nonfatal fractures prevent people from ever again walking without assistance. (And of course, you can forget about fun things like skiing.)

But osteoporosis is preventable, and even those who already suffer from it can both slow down the rate at which they lose bone mass and increase their resistance to fractures. "Osteoporosis need not be an inevitable part of aging," says William A. Peck, M.D., founding president of the National Osteoporosis Foundation (NOF).

The first step in protecting yourself, say the experts, is knowing the causes. This will also help you determine how to prevent or treat osteoporosis—including whether to use hormone replacement therapy or other medications that can lessen bone loss.

## WHO GETS OSTEOPOROSIS, AND WHY?

Most of us think of our bones as solid, permanent structures. But bone is dynamic, continually breaking down and building up anew throughout our lives.

All of us begin to lose bone after we reach our early to mid 30s, the age at which we achieve what scientists call peak bone mass. Our skeletons will never be denser or stronger. From that point on, we gradually lose bone density at a rate of about 3 percent per decade.

In women, that loss speeds up dramatically just after menopause, when the rate of bone loss can reach *3 to 5 percent a year*. Luckily, bone loss slows after the first five years following menopause to about 1 percent a year, according to Robert Heaney, M.D., professor of medicine at Creighton University School of Medicine in Omaha and a leading expert on osteoporosis.

Women often lose bone rapidly after menopause because their production of estrogen plummets, and this hormone—like the male hormone testosterone—is essential to protect bone tissue. Though women continue to produce small quantities of estrogen after menopause, these amounts are often inadequate to maintain healthy bone.

Men also suffer from osteoporosis, but far fewer of them than women: Only one-eighth as many men get this disease, and it occurs about a decade later than in women. Since men have a shorter life expectancy that women, many of them die before ever manifesting osteoporosis. Men don't suffer the hormone drop that women do in menopause, and they usually have much greater bone mass to start with. Men who have low testosterone levels or experience a drop in testosterone as they age, however, are advised to have testosterone replacement therapy to protect their bones, says Maria Fiatarone, M.D., chief of the physiology laboratory at the U.S. Department of Agriculture's (USDA) Human Nutrition Research Center on Aging at Tufts University in Boston and assistant professor in the division on aging at Harvard Medical School.

Many factors influence bone loss, like exercise and good nutrition. "Lifestyle has a huge amount to do with how much this disease affects you," says Bess Dawson-Hughes, M.D., chief of the calcium and bone metabolism laboratory at Tufts University.

### BONE BOOSTING BEGINS WITH CALCIUM

Calcium is one of the most important nutrients involved in building bones, but intake of this mineral has dropped significantly since 1950, says Dr. Heaney. "And on the whole, modern humans get far less than our primitive ancestors. We don't eat the greens and roots that they ate, and even our milk consumption is down now," he says.

Fortunately, there are so many good sources of calcium that even vegetarians and people who avoid milk products can get more than enough to meet their needs. The Recommended Dietary Allowance is 800 milligrams for men and 1,000 milligrams for women. In addition, the National Osteoporosis Foundation suggests 1,000 to 1,500 milligrams of calcium daily for men and women over the age of 64; 1,200 to 1,600 milligrams for pregnant or nursing women; 1,500 milligrams for menopausal women who do not take estrogen; and 1,000 milligrams for women who do take estrogen.

How do you know if you're getting enough calcium? Each serving of dairy food provides roughly 250 milligrams of calcium, so if you reach for three or four a day, you'll get 900 to 1,200 milligrams. Among the best sources of this mineral are:

- low-fat and nonfat dairy products, including yogurt
- green vegetables, such as collard greens, bok choy, broccoli, kale and turnip greens (but not spinach—it's rich in oxalic acid, which blocks calcium absorption)

- tofu and soybean products
- fish, including canned salmon, sardines and mackerel, when both flesh and bones are eaten
- almonds
- cereals fortified with calcium
- orange juice fortified with calcium
- calcium supplements, especially when calcium-rich foods are not consumed regularly

Women especially should eat lots of calcium-rich foods throughout their lives, but they should be particularly aware of their calcium needs in their 30s and 40s. "The idea is for women to go into menopause with as much bone as possible," says Dr. Heaney.

Don't exclude other nutrients from your bone-building plan; vitamin D is essential to help your body use calcium. "People who do not get outdoors, or older people who are shut-ins or who live in nursing homes, often fail to get the sunlight and vitamin D they need," says Robert Lang, M.D., an endocrinologist and expert on osteoporosis in New Haven, Connecticut. Just five to ten minutes in sunlight each day will give you all the vitamin D your body needs, without increasing your risk of skin cancer. Or you can get your D by eating oily fish such as tuna and salmon, egg yolks and fortified milk. Other foods— including baby foods, breakfast cereal, bread, pasta, rice and oils—may have vitamin D added as well.

### DEM BONES: USE 'EM OR LOSE 'EM

All weight-bearing exercise makes bones denser and stronger—and lack of exercise means bone loss. "The more demands you make on your body in the form of exercise, the more bone you produce. Cut back on exercise, and you cut back on bone," explains Dr. Heaney.

"Exercise can combat osteoporosis by slowing bone loss," says Roger Fielding, exercise physiologist at the USDA's Human Nutrition Research Center on Aging at Tufts University. "People who engage in hard work or some form of resistance training show greater bone density. You see denser bones in lumberjacks, for example. In tennis players, you find that the bones in the racket arm are denser than in the non-racket arm."

Not only does exercise strengthen bones and muscles, it may also prevent falls that can lead to fractures. "People who exercise tend to have better balance and walk better and therefore may not be as susceptible to falls and broken bones," Fielding says. Here's how to make the most of bone-building workouts.

**Choose your exercises.** The ideal program includes aerobic exercises, such as brisk walking, plus some form of resistance training with weights, say scientists at the research center. It's best to choose exercises that focus on the areas of your body most susceptible to fracture: legs, hips, wrists and arms.

**Work out regularly.** For best results, the Tufts researchers recommend that people work out for about 45 minutes, three to four times a week, doing 3 sets of resistance exercises, with 8 to 10 repetitions per set.

**Find your capacity.** "If you lift weights, you should work out at 80 percent of your maximum weight-lifting capacity," says Fielding. To do that, you'll have to find the maximum weight you can lift once, then work out with a weight that is 80 percent of that. If your maximum is 100 pounds, you should work out with 80 pounds. If you can only lift 50 pounds once, work out with 40.

**Join a gym.** A gym membership gives you access to weight machines that allow you to do resistance exercises without worrying about dropping free weights on a foot or a leg. Some university health clubs, fitness centers and gyms have programs designed for people on fixed incomes.

**Stick with it.** One important factor in a successful exercise program is consistency. "Bone growth is a fairly slow process," says Fielding. "You need about a year to make significant improvement in bone density. That's a lot different than what you get from muscles and the heart, which improve much faster."

## HOW TO WORK OUT AT HOME

You can do these exercises at home using small hand-held free weights; ankle and wrist weights; resistance bands, which look like oversize elastic bands; or exercise tubes, a variation on the elastic-band theme. Or you can use a bicycle inner tube, and partially fill bleach bottles with sand or water to use as weights.

Remember not to hurry or jerk your body, and keep your back straight. Repeat the movements 8 to 12 times to make up 1 set. If possible, do 3 sets of each exercise.

**Chest pull.** Using a resistance band or exercise tube, stand with your feet shoulder-width apart and extend your arms in front. Pull your arms apart, stretching the band. Bring your arms back slowly.

**Outer thigh lift.** Using an elastic band wrapped around your ankles, lie on your side with your legs straight. Lift your upper leg until the band is taut. Lower your leg slowly. Roll over on your other side and repeat with your other leg.

**Outer thigh press.** Lie on your back, with an elastic band around your ankles and your hands under your buttocks. Lift both legs into the air, and press them apart until the band is taut. Slowly bring your legs together.

**Standing arm row.** Stand with an elastic band looped beneath one or both feet, while holding the ends in your hands. Pull your fists up toward your underarms. Lower your fists slowly, then slowly pull the band up toward your shoulders, in a rowing action. Slowly allow the band to recoil. Repeat.

**Lateral raises.** Stand, and lift a hand-held weight from your side until it is parallel with the floor, so that your arm forms a 90-degree angle with your body. Slowly let the weight return to your side. Repeat, alternating arms.

**Triceps press.** Lift a hand-held weight straight up above your head, and slowly bring it back down behind your head. Repeat.

**Biceps curl.** Hold a hand-weight in front of your body and curl it to your chest, keeping your elbow at your hip. Repeat.

**Chair push-up.** Place a chair with its back against a wall. Kneel in front of the chair, grip the chair seat, and do a push-up against the chair. Repeat.

## PRACTICE MODERATION FOR STRONGER BONES

Some scientists suggest that changing certain habits can help contribute to good bone health. In any case, moderating your intake of these substances can't hurt.

**Cut back on booze.** "A number of studies have shown that hip fractures are more common in male and female alcoholics than in their nonalcoholic peers," says Ariel Simkin, Ph.D., coauthor with Judith Ayalon of *Bone-Loading, the New Way to Prevent and Combat the Thinning Bones of Osteoporosis.*

"Alcohol is one of the major risk factors for osteoporosis," says Dr. Lang. Alcohol may alter the hormonal balance needed for strong bones (and may also promote calcium loss in urine).

**Toss the cigarettes.** To alcohol, add that old health nemesis, smoking. Women who smoke tend to reach menopause earlier than nonsmoking women, which may be one of the ways that smoking predisposes them to earlier signs of osteoporosis.

**Steer clear of diet culprits.** Consuming high amounts of protein, salt, caffeine and phosphates, which are commonly found in cola beverages and coffee, have all been linked to increased calcium losses from bone. "Excesses of these nutrients tend to cause problems for people who have dietary extremes, like protein fanatics," says Dr. Dawson-Hughes. "As long as you're eating a healthy diet and moderate amounts of these foods, you're not likely to experience a problem."

## WEIGHING THE BENEFITS OF HORMONES

Once a woman passes menopause and loses most of her ability to produce estrogen, she must either rely upon her existing bone reserves or take hormone replacement therapy (HRT) or other medications to slow the loss of bone. "A woman can lose as much as 15 percent of her skeleton during those first five years after menopause," says Dr. Dawson-Hughes. "The treatment goal is to slow that rate of bone loss, which estrogen does." (HRT also usually includes progesterone, another hormone.)

# CONSIDER YOUR MEDICATIONS

Certain drugs accelerate bone loss, cautions Maria Fiatarone, M.D., chief of the physiology laboratory at the U.S. Department of Agriculture's Human Nutrition Research Center on Aging at Tufts University in Boston and assistant professor in the division on aging at Harvard Medical School. These include:

- Thyroid hormone replacement
- Prednisone
- Dilantin

Individuals taking these drugs should take the following measures to help protect their skeleton.

1. Check with the doctor to make sure you are on the *lowest possible* dosage of your prescribed medication.
2. In the case of prednisone and Dilantin, take supplemental vitamin D in the amount of 800 international units per day. This is twice the amount in a standard multivitamin pill, so you'll need a separate supplement.
3. Take 1,000 milligrams of calcium daily.

Still, the decision to take HRT is not clear-cut. "Many factors weigh in the decision to take estrogen," says Dr. Heaney. One is the risk of breast cancer: Some studies show an increased risk of the cancer in women who took estrogen, while others do not.

According to Frank Sacks, M.D., of Harvard Medical School, "a consensus analysis of all the studies shows that it isn't clear whether there is an increased risk. If there is a risk, it's slight."

Regardless, if breast disease runs in your family, HRT may not be for you. "Breast cancer is prevalent now," says Dr. Heaney, "so you have to take into consideration the family history and whether a woman is at higher risk of the illness."

When taken alone, estrogen may increase the risk of uterine

cancer, say the authors of *Bone-Loading*. Fortunately, the risk can be cut considerably by taking progesterone as well.

Dr. Simkin, a senior researcher at the Jerusalem Osteoporosis Center, Hadassah University Hospital in Jerusalem, Israel, and Ayalon, a physiotherapist at the Wingate Institute for Physical Education and Sport, also in Jerusalem, are convinced that it's best to combine exercise and increased calcium intake with hormone therapy, allowing the dosage of estrogen to be reduced. Estrogen doses have also been cut in half in the last 15 years, which significantly reduces any risk.

On the pro side, some studies show that women who take estrogen live longer than those who do not. And estrogen significantly reduces a woman's chances of developing heart disease. "The possible harmful effects related to breast cancer are nowhere near as great as the beneficial protection from heart disease," says Dr. Sacks.

"You have to explain all the risks to a woman," says Dr. Dawson-Hughes, "and then let her decide." She urges that women who fall into the high-risk category—especially those who have small skeletons or experience early menopause—have a bone-density test before they make a decision.

## AN ALTERNATIVE TO ESTROGEN REPLACEMENT

Meanwhile, other medications such as calcitonin may help slow the rate of bone-density loss, even among women who do not take estrogens. Calcitonin, a hormone extracted from salmon, is currently given by injection, but a nasal spray is pending approval from the Food and Drug Administration (FDA). "People with a high bone turnover respond nicely to calcitonin," says Dr. Dawson-Hughes.

Other drugs are also being tested by the FDA. "We're going to see a lot of new research coming out on osteoporosis in the very near future," says Dr. Sacks. "A lot of the questions that linger now will be answered."

## ANTI-AGING CHECKUP
# ASK ABOUT A BONE TEST

The best way to determine if you are at risk for osteoporosis is to have a bone density analysis. The next best thing is to know whether you fall into the high-risk group. Answer Yes or No to the questions in the following summary of risk factors.

_____ Are you over 55? The risk of contracting osteoporosis increases as you get older.

_____ Are you female? Women are more likely than men to get the disease and suffer more fractures.

_____ Are you of Asian or Caucasian descent? Fair-skinned and fair-haired people suffer higher rates of osteoporosis than darker people.

_____ Did you start menopause before age 50?

_____ Do you have small, thin bones?

_____ Do you have an endocrine disease or metabolic disorder such as diabetes, thyroid disease, chronic renal failure or hyperactivity? (These diseases are associated with greater risk of osteoporosis.)

_____ Do you take corticosteroids such as prednisone or other drugs for allergies, arthritis and inflammatory diseases?

_____ Are you sedentary and get little exercise?

_____ Do you eat few dairy products?

_____ Do you seldom get out in the sun? (A lack of vitamin D is linked to osteoporosis.)

_____ Do you smoke or consume large amounts of alcohol or caffeine?

_____ Have any of your female relatives ever suffered from osteoporosis-related fractures of the hip, spine, waist, ribs or pelvis?

### INTERPRETING YOUR ANSWERS

If you answered Yes to more than one of these questions, you should talk to your physician about your potential risk for osteoporosis and begin taking measures now to protect your bones from damage in the future.

# 27

# OVERWEIGHT

### Painless Ways to Ditch
### Those Extra Pounds

**We're** a nation obsessed with size and weight loss. But many of us do carry extra pounds. Typically, Americans gain a pound or two a year after they reach adulthood. By the age of 35 or 45, many folks find themselves several sizes larger than they were at 21.

"Overweight is a big problem in the United States," says Kelly Brownell, Ph.D., professor of psychology at Yale University and a top obesity researcher. Nearly two-thirds of U.S. adults are overweight, according to a 1990 nationwide survey conducted by Louis Harris and Associates.

What's wrong with that extra weight? Chances are, you don't feel or look your best with a spare tire around your middle. But more significantly, being overweight increases your chances of suffering heart disease; adult-onset diabetes; high blood pressure; gallstones; rectal, colon, breast and prostate cancers; and complications after surgery.

Safely losing excess weight—and keeping it off—is one of the best ways to retain vitality and cut disease risks. Trimming your weight mows down numerous risk factors in one swoop. In laboratory studies, animals fed fewer calories live nearly a third longer than their plumper peers, and they have fewer cancerous tumors and other signs of disease. "If everybody in the United States maintained their ideal weight, the incidence of Type II diabetes would be greatly reduced, hypertension would be much less common and so would coronary disease," says Meir Stampfer, M.D., Dr.P.H., associate professor of epidemiology at Harvard School of Public Health.

Losing weight too quickly or by extremely low-calorie or liquid diets—or letting your weight yo-yo up and down—can be harmful to your health, however. Weight loss must be a slow process and requires a commitment to healthy eating patterns and moderate exercise. Here's how to design your own painless, at-home weight-loss program.

## CREATE A FIGURE-FRIENDLY MENU

Want to lose weight, but you can't stand being hungry? You don't have to suffer to shed fat. Follow these guidelines, and you'll soon discover that you have plenty of tasty, good-for-you options to quiet a grumbling tummy.

**Load up on carbohydrates.** Garth Fisher, Ph.D., and his colleagues at Brigham Young University in Provo, Utah, put 26 overweight women on diets. One group was allowed to eat all the grains, vegetables and fruits they desired, while the other group was restricted to 800 calories a day.

After 16 weeks, all the dieters lost weight, more than 13 pounds on average. But the group on the restricted diet complained of lack of energy and being hungry and anxious, while the others weren't troubled by hunger. So instead of starving yourself, reach for nourishing and satisfying complex carbohydrates. These include fruits, vegetables and whole grains, such as brown rice, oatmeal, barley and whole-wheat bread.

**Limit fats.** Fat, the most calorically dense food, adds more calories than you can burn off by normal metabolism. Consequently, the fat you eat gets deposited on your hips, thighs or elsewhere on your body. You need to limit how many fat-filled foods you eat, steering clear of fatty meats such as sausages and many lunch meats, butter, sour cream, salad dressings, mayonnaise, ice cream, chocolate and nuts. Crackers, chips and cheese can also be high in fat, so check the labels.

This doesn't mean you have to give up your favorite foods completely; just reserve them for special treats. You can also cut fat by reaching for low-fat or skim milk and using low-fat or nonfat versions of dressings, cheese, yogurt and sour cream.

Nonfat foods are the fastest growing segment of the supermarket industry, and these products taste 1,000 percent better than early ventures into "diet food." Substituting healthier choices should be a breeze.

**Scrutinize those labels.** Ideally, fat will make up no more than 25 percent of what you eat. Here's an easy way to insure that prepared foods have less than 25 percent of their calories in fat.

1. Find the total calories listed on the label, and drop the last digit of that number. (If an oatmeal cookie contains 163 calories, drop the last digit to get the number 16.)
2. Divide that number by 4. (16 divided by 4 is 4.)
3. Compare that final number with the grams of fat listed on the label. If it's more than the number you just came up with, the food contains more than 25 percent of its calories in fat.

**Fill up with fiber.** A high-fiber diet fills you up but not out. "Fiber creates an appetite-suppressing effect," says nutritionist Diane Grabowski, R.D., of the Pritikin Longevity Center in Santa Monica, California. "It keeps you satisfied longer, so you don't feel the need to cheat on your diet." Added benefits are that fiber also assists in digestion and regularity and may lower your cholesterol level and protect against colon cancer.

High-fiber foods include whole grains as well as most vegetables and fruits and legumes such as beans, lentils, chickpeas and split peas. Breakfast foods such as whole-grain pancakes, muffins and cereals are also loaded with fiber.

**Explore herbs and spices.** Fat is tasty, no doubt about it. So when you cut back, you may find your food tastes a bit bland. Try seasoning with such delicious herbs as cilantro, basil, leeks, onions, shallots, parsley and garlic—they're just the beginning of a new adventure in cooking. Sprinkle lemon juice on salads and steamed vegetables.

**Treat yourself to breakfast.** While you sleep, your body slows down and you burn calories at a much slower rate. It isn't until you wake up, start moving around and eat breakfast that your metabolism kicks into gear again. Skipping the morning meal keeps your metabolism at a sluggish pace, and the lack of fuel means that you're more likely to overeat later in the day.

"Beginning the day with a healthy breakfast actually gives you the energy to perform at your peak all day long," says James M. Rippe, M.D., director of the exercise, physiology and nutrition laboratory at the University of Massachusetts Medical Center in Worcester.

**Bid adieu to booze.** As everyone with a beer belly knows, drinking alcohol slows down weight loss. The body tends to store the extra calories from alcohol as fat, according to a study published in the *New England Journal of Medicine*. The researchers found that the alcohol prevented fat from being oxidized, or burned as fuel, resulting in weight gain.

## REV UP YOUR ENGINE

"It's had to reduce your weight by controlling calories alone. If you exercise as well, you're more likely to be able to maintain the weight loss," says Dr. Stampfer. Regular exercise speeds up your metabolism not only when you're working out but also while you're resting. Exercise builds muscle, and muscle burns more calories than fat. So the more muscle you have, the more your body is consuming calories. That makes exercise one of the best weight-controlling tools you have, especially after age 35, when your metabolism begins to slow down—unless you continue to exercise regularly. (Exercise also lowers blood pressure, relieves stress and helps keep your heart healthy.)

You don't have to run marathons to benefit from exercise: A little goes a long way. "I think that exercise should not be looked upon as doing something until it hurts," says Maria Simonson, Ph.D., Sc.D., director of the Health, Weight and Stress Clinic at the Johns Hopkins Medical Institutions in Baltimore. All you have to do is get out there and move. Try walking, ballroom dancing, bicycling, rowing, stair climbing, almost anything that gets your limbs moving and your heart pumping a little. (See chapters 1, 13 and 32.)

Strength training can also speed metabolism and prevent the shift from muscle to fat. "A resistance-training program is good for 35-plus looks, too," explains George Blackburn,

M.D., Ph.D., chief of the nutrition/metabolism laboratory at New England Deaconess Hospital in Boston and associate professor of medicine at Harvard Medical School. "If you've lost your muscle tone, lifting weights will help you get it back, and if you do resistance exercise consistently, you won't lose it. Look for a well-supervised program where they have experience with over-35 clients, and talk to your doctor before you start." If you're over 40, get medical approval before increasing exercise levels or taking on a new form of activity, especially if you have a chronic illness.

## THINK POSITIVELY

The road to weight loss can be a bumpy one, and it affects much more than the outer you—your spirits will be subjected to plenty of ups and downs, too. When you find yourself in a valley, the following suggestions might give you a lift.

**Jot down your thoughts.** Your health and weight are a direct extension of your thoughts and feelings. By becoming conscious of how you think and how you use food to deal with problems and emotions, you can learn to control the urges that lead to compulsive eating. Herbert Benson, M.D., associate professor of medicine at Harvard Medical School, urges you to recognize when, where and why you overeat. Is it a certain time? A certain place? Are you feeling lonely or bored?

Write these things down, and after a few days look over your log. Try to figure out at what point in the chain of events you can break the pattern and change the outcome. Perhaps you could take a brisk walk or call a friend instead of reaching for cookies, or fulfill your urge to crunch with carrot sticks or plain popcorn. Try this strategy the next time you find yourself wanting to eat when you aren't hungry. If it doesn't work at first, keep trying.

**Appreciate your food.** We all tend to eat quickly and unconsciously. The next time you eat, take a few deep breaths before beginning. Try to truly enjoy your meals, rather than gulping them down. (And *don't* eat in front of the television!) The secret is to savor each mouthful of food with all your senses. You'll eventually be satisfied sooner and with less food.

**Be patient.** You didn't gain weight overnight; you won't lose it overnight. "For permanent weight control, losing a half-pound to a pound a week is plenty," says Ronette L. Kolotkin, Ph.D., director of behavioral programs at the Duke University Diet and Fitness Center in Durham, North Carolina. "Quick fixes never work. If you're not ready to give it time, you're not ready to lose weight."

**Don't be too hard on yourself.** "Preparing to lose weight means realizing that everyone makes mistakes. Forgive yourself," says Arizona weight-loss psychologist Susan Olson, Ph.D., director of psychological services at the Southwest Bariatric Nutrition Center in Tempe, Arizona. Overeating one day doesn't mean that you can't eat sensibly the next.

And don't try to lead a Spartan existence with no treats of favorite foods. If going out for an ice-cream cone on Saturday night satisfies your sweet tooth and allows you to eat more healthful foods all week without feeling deprived, then enjoy that cone, and don't worry about it.

---

### ANTI-AGING CHECKUP
## BEFORE TACKLING WEIGHT LOSS, CHECK OUT YOUR PERSONALITY TYPE

Certain techniques might be right on target with your own personality traits, habits and strengths, while the same approach may do nothing for another person—or even cause him or her to eat *more*. To find out which approach is best suited to your own needs and lifestyle, answer the following questions Yes or No.

**PART A**

_____ 1. Do you like to move your furniture around and redecorate?

_____ 2. Do you frequently try new hobbies?

_____ 3. Do changes that dismay others at work just seem like welcome challenges to you?

*continued*

____ 4. Do you enjoy new, unfamiliar foods and schedules when traveling?

**PART B**

____ 1. Do you thrive on schedules and routine?
____ 2. Do you pay all your bills on time?
____ 3. Do you pay your taxes by March?
____ 4. Do you keep an extensive list of telephone numbers at hand and a marked-up calendar?

**PART C**

____ 1. Do you love to get to the bottom of things?
____ 2. Do you want your mechanic to explain in detail what is wrong with your car?
____ 3. If you run across a question you can't answer, do you research the topic until you find out?
____ 4. When your checkbook doesn't balance by a few cents, do you painstakingly check each entry to find the error?

**PART D**

____ 1. Do you frequently fantasize about future accomplishments?
____ 2. Are you deeply inspired by people who succeeded in their goals despite enormous odds?
____ 3. Do you believe you can accomplish anything you set your mind to?
____ 4. Are you optimistic that projects you begin will turn out well?

## INTERPRETING YOUR ANSWERS

**Part A:** Mostly Yes answers to these questions means you will have better success at weight loss by heeding these tips.

- Don't try to stick with one program for a long time, especially if it's highly regimented. Choose a program that allows ample freedom of choice, substitution and experimentation.

*continued*

- After a month or so, feel free to try new foods, recipes, exercises or mental-reinforcement techniques.
- Your enthusiasm may tempt you to cut back too drastically on your food intake—don't do it.
- Try eating dinner with your fork in your opposite hand (left if you're right-handed and vice versa).

**Part B:** If you answered Yes to these questions, consider the following idea.

- Because you're well organized, you should be able to shop from a list. Allow yourself one or two planned treats.
- Eat only at scheduled times in scheduled places. Most overeating occurs in the kitchen and in front of the TV.
- Don't eat foods from their original containers. You'll usually wind up eating more than you do when you serve a measured portion and eat from a plate.
- Eat a relatively large breakfast and a good lunch every day. This habit can result in significant weight loss even when your total calories remain the same.
- Play slow, classical music whenever you sit down to eat. You'll eat more slowly, consume less and enjoy your meal more.

**Part C:** If you answered Yes to these questions, you'll benefit by following these tips.

- Figure out all the reasons you want to lose weight.
- Keep a food diary, writing down everything you eat and drink, when and where you ate it and how you felt.
- Determine the times you eat when you're not really hungry or when you overeat, and devise ways to steer clear of food at these times.
- Look around your home for food "triggers"—candy dishes in the living room or a box of crackers on your desk—and put these items away.

*continued*

**Part D:** If these questions describe you, here are some tips to help you acquire healthy eating habits.

- Use your talent for positive thinking to get yourself past food cravings.
- Congratulate yourself every day that you eat sensibly.
- Set a reasonable, sensible, long-term goal.
- Frequently imagine yourself with the extra weight gone.
- Make "goals" for your exercise, and keep a log of miles walked or minutes spent weight lifting.

*Editor's note:* Certain weight-loss tips, of course, apply no matter what your personality type. Some across-the-board advice: Take up a sensible exercise program, choose low-fat and nonfat products, reduce "empty" calories such as soda and alcoholic beverages, and fill up on plenty of whole grains, fruits and vegetables.

# 28

# PROSTATE PROBLEMS

## What Goes Wrong (and Why)

**The** prostate gland might be described as modern man's Achilles' heel. Virtually every man over 50 can expect to experience swelling of the gland, which can lead to simple discomfort or serious complications and disease.

Located just beneath the bladder, the prostate produces fluid that keeps sperm healthy and mobile. The prostate gland is about the size of a chestnut, with the urethra—the tube that carries urine from the bladder to the tip of the penis—passing directly through the middle of it. (Think of a small doughnut, with a straw going through the hole.) The urethra also has tiny ducts that can block urine and allow sperm to pass during ejaculation.

According to the experts, every man over the age of 50 has some swelling, called benign prostatic hyperplasia (BPH), in his prostate gland. In many cases, it's harmless, but the enlargement can cause problems when the swelling clamps down on the urethra, sometimes blocking the flow of urine. "All men undergo some tissue expansion," says Cliff Vestal, M.D., a urologist at the University of Colorado Health Sciences Center in Denver. "But only a percentage of men will experience symptoms of BPH or prostate cancer."

## WHEN THINGS GO AWRY

Why does the prostate enlarge? "We don't really know," says Robert P. Hubern, M.D., chief of urologic oncology at Roswell Park Cancer Institute in Buffalo. "Most researchers think that a hormone triggers this unwarranted growth. But we don't have enough solid evidence to say more than it happens as you age, and there doesn't seem to be a way to stop it." The hormone in question is dihydrotestosterone, a product of testosterone metabolism.

For perhaps three out of ten men with prostate problems, the symptoms simply disappear spontaneously or yield to minor drug treatment, says Dr. Vestal.

Prostate enlargement and the resultant signs of urinary obstruction generally occur after age 50. For younger men who experience difficulty urinating, the problem is usually infection of the prostate—bacterial prostatitis, or swelling of the prostate.

The prostate can become infected at any age, however. The infection usually starts in the bladder and spreads via the urethra. Symptoms may include difficulty urinating, fever and pain in the lower abdomen and the back of the legs. "Quinolones, which are broad-spectrum antibiotics, are currently considered the best drugs for the job," says Christopher M. Dixon, M.D., assistant professor of urology at the Medical College of Wisconsin—Milwaukee. "In most cases, symptoms improve in 24 to 48 hours, but it may take two to three weeks to resolve the infection completely."

## THE PRIME SUSPECT: DIET

The major lifestyle factor that may encourage the development of the disease is diet, especially one high in fat and low in beta-carotene, a nutrient in many vegetables that converts to vitamin A in the body. A diet high in fat—especially animal fat—may affect the hormonal balance within a man's prostate and increase the level of dihydrotestosterone, according to a report in the *American Journal of Epidemiology*. Other dietary factors that may cause the prostate to swell include cigarette smoking and excessive alcohol consumption. Here's what you can do to protect your prostate.

**Cut back on fat.** After reviewing numerous studies, researchers at the Kuakini Medical Canter in Honolulu say that data points to dietary fat as a key danger, specifically animal fat and saturated fat.

The researchers speculate that dietary fat changes hormonal balances in men, as it does in women. When both white and black men switch to vegetarian diets, the few hormones are released in the urine. The researchers theorize that dietary fat may change the internal hormonal balance of the sex organs. So it seems prudent for every man to heed the advice of the U.S. Surgeon General and the National Cancer Institute and reduce his level of fat intake, especially saturated fat.

**Chow down on beta-carotene.** Animal studies show that beta-carotene may block the onset of cancer at several places, including the prostate. While numerous studies of human populations support this theory, other research has failed to show this effect. But research has consistently shown beta-carotene's influence in enhancing immunity, including its ability to help prevent certain cancers—so it's wise to increase your intake of this nutrient.

**Give these metals a miss.** Cadmium and other heavy metals are known to depress the immune system and they may well play a role in the onset of prostate cancer, says Dr. Vestal. Research suggests cadmium exposure on the job or from smoking may increase the risk of prostate cancer.

## THE STRESSED-OUT PROSTATE

Some physicians estimate that 95 percent of all chronic cases of prostatitis are stress-related. "Usually men with chronic prostatitis live high-stress lifestyles," says Richard Schmidt, M.D., professor of urology and director of neurourology at the University of Colorado Health Science Center. Dr. Schmidt notes that people react to stress in various ways. Some get migraines, some get low-back pain, and some concentrate their tension on their lower pelvic muscles and the prostate gland. When the pelvic muscles are too tense, they prevent adequate urination, which can reduce flow. "Over time, urine backs up into the prostatic ducts, which causes the chronic inflammation and pain," says Dr. Schmidt. Try these suggestions to stop the stress.

**Calm down.** In some cases, muscle relaxants or hot baths will ease the tension and restore health. (See chapter 59.) Some physicians recommend frequent ejaculation to relax the muscles and drain the gland.

**Relax your muscles.** Dr. Schmidt says the best method is to learn to relax the pelvic-floor muscles consciously whenever urinating. With a little concentration or the help of a urologist, men can learn to identify and relax their pelvic-floor muscles, either by visualization or with the assistance of biofeedback.

## CLUES TO CANCER PREVENTION

Prostate cancer is the most common cancer occurring in American men and the second-leading cancer killer of men. An estimated 122,000 American men get prostate cancer each year, and 32,000 die from it. Though the average age of men who contract prostate cancer is 70, all men over 40 are at risk.

This disease offers up a host of mysteries that researchers have yet to solve. For example, the incidence of the disease varies widely according to race and geographical location. In the U.S., about 1 in 11 white men and 1 in 9 black men develop prostate cancer, while the disease is rare in Asians.

And immigrants to the United States suffer higher rates of prostate cancer than do their countrymen at home. Poles in their native land, for example, rarely get prostate cancer, but those who emigrate to the United States are just as apt to get the disease as Americans. Likewise, Japanese men in Japan have a very low rate of prostate cancer, but when they move to the United States, their odds of getting the disease increase fourfold.

What experts *do* know about prostate cancer is that tests to detect it include a digital rectal examination, in which a doctor feels the prostate through the rectum and assesses its condition. Next, the doctor is likely to order a blood test called a prostate specific antigen (PSA) test, which will detect the level of glycoprotein being produced by the prostate. (All prostates produce the protein, but as the gland enlarges, it produces more.) A score of less than 4 micrograms per liter is normal; readings above 4 call for further tests to determine whether a man has BPH or cancer, says Dr. Vestal.

"There are detectable increases even in the early stages of tumor growth," says T. Ming Chu, Ph.D., developer of the PSA test and chairman of diagnostic immunology research at Roswell Park Cancer Institute. "That can give the patient a head start on treatment once the diagnosis is confirmed."

A PSA test is inexpensive and easy, but it isn't perfect. "In up to one-half of men with known early prostate cancer, the PSA can be normal, and one-third of men with benign prostate disease may have an elevated PSA level but not have prostate cancer," says Richard D. Williams, M.D., chairman of the urology department at the University of Iowa in Iowa City.

If the digital rectal exam and PSA test suggest a problem, a doctor will likely order an ultrasound and, if necessary, a needle biopsy.

---

### ANTI-AGING CHECKUP
## SIGNS OF A PROBLEM PROSTATE

Answer the following questions Yes or No.

\_\_\_\_ Do you have blood in your urine?
\_\_\_\_ Do you regularly get up three or more times a night to urinate?
\_\_\_\_ Do you urinate frequently during the day?
\_\_\_\_ Do you have trouble starting urine flow or stopping it?
\_\_\_\_ Do you have repeated burning or stinging pain during urination?

### INTERPRETING YOUR ANSWERS

Only your doctor can tell you the exact condition of your prostate, so if you answered Yes to any of these questions, you should check with him or her.

# 29

# SEX

### Enhance the Intimate Side of Your Life

**You're** a bit older, perhaps a bit grayer, perhaps a bit heavier. But that certainly doesn't mean your love life is over.

Duke University researchers have found that eight out of ten men in their late 60s continue to be sexually active, while one in four men 78 and older continue to be sexually involved. Women, too, retain their sex drive and interest throughout life, and decreases in sexual activity among older women often occur simply because they have no partners.

Physical changes do occur as you age, but none of them need undermine the pleasures of a couple's sex life. In fact, many older people maintain that sex is *better* in later years because there are no worries of pregnancy, no children nearby and no pressures of work.

### KEEPING YOUR SEX LIFE YOUNG

Here are some ways to enliven or revitalize your sex life.

**Take your time.** As both men and women age, sexual response slows down a bit. Women's ovaries produce less estrogen after menopause, which causes the lining of the vagina to become thinner and to secrete less lubricating mucus during sexual arousal. This means she may need longer to be ready to make love or may want to use a lubricating jelly. Men secrete less testosterone as they age, so erections take longer to develop and may be less firm. All this means is that making love may take a bit longer than it used to.

**Rule out medical causes.** In women, a bladder infection or yeast infection—easily curable with medication—can make intercourse uncomfortable or even painful. (See chapter 5.) In men, many medical problems can cause impotence, including diabetes, Parkinson's disease, liver or kidney disease and lowerback problems. So the first step with love-making difficulties is a visit to your physician.

**Check out your medication.** As much as one-fourth of sexual impotence is caused by medication, physicians estimate. Hypertension drugs, particularly thiazide diuretics, and tranquilizers cause most of the problems. But antidepressants, antihistamines, antispasmodics, heart regulators and ulcer medications can also cause impotence.

**Control your blood pressure—naturally.** Trading in your easy chair for an exercycle and making other healthful lifestyle changes can pump up the sex drive as well as control blood pressure, according to one study. Researchers divided 79 men with high blood pressure into three groups: One took the antihypertensive drug propranolol, one took a placebo pill, and a third began a program of exercise, improved diet and stress management. The lifestyle changes of the third group not only lowered blood pressure but also heightened sexual arousal and pleasure.

"This is the first time we've shown that lowering blood pressure by lifestyle changes in and of itself improves sex life," says John B. Kostis, M.D., chairman of the department of medicine at the University of Medicine and Dentistry of New Jersey, Robert Wood Johnson Medical School in New Brunswick. (Don't, of course, reduce your medication or stop taking it without instructions from your doctor.)

**Get a workout.** Getting out of bed may help boost a man's performance *in* bed. A group of 78 previously inactive but healthy men jogged or bicycled at 75 to 80 percent of their aerobic capacity for an hour a day, 3½ days a week, while a control group of 17 men didn't exercise. After nine months, the exercisers reported a 30 percent increase in frequency of intercourse, with 26 percent more orgasms and more caressing and passionate kissing. In contrast, the nonexercisers had sex slightly *less* often.

## ANTI-AGING CHECKUP
# WHEN THE SPARK HAS FIZZLED

So you can't get your spouse interested in sex, or perhaps your own desire has flickered out. You may have just fallen out of the habit because of lack of time, the arrival of children in the household and increasing work pressures—in which case you may be able to easily light the flame again with time and some romantic effort.

But there's a big difference between not being in the mood for sex and not being able to *have* sex, says William Young, M.D., of the Masters and Johnson Institute in St. Louis—and one of you may have a problem that makes sex difficult or impossible. The problem could be psychological, physical or a combination of the two. Answer these key questions Yes or No to help pinpoint the cause.

### FOR WOMEN
_____ 1. Are you urinating more often than usual?
_____ 2. Do you have an abnormal vaginal discharge?
_____ 3. Do you feel pain deep within the vagina during intercourse?
_____ 4. Does your vagina feel dry and tight?
_____ 5. Is penetration difficult or impossible?
_____ 6. Are you unable to reach orgasm?

### FOR MEN
_____ 7. Do you get an erection, but cannot sustain it long enough to satisfy your partner? Or do you never get an erection?
_____ 8. Do you have pain in your penis during intercourse?
_____ 9. Do you have pain when you ejaculate?
____ 10. Is the tip of your penis sore after intercourse?

### INTERPRETING YOUR ANSWERS

1. You may have cystitis or a bladder infection.
2. You may have a vaginal infection.

*continued*

3. There can be various causes for this, including endometriosis, an ovarian cyst or a tipped uterus.
4. This could be caused by anxiety or a decline in estrogen levels.
5. This could signal vaginismus, in which there's an involuntary tightening of the muscles surrounding the vagina and the outer third of the vagina closes.
6. There could be any of a number of causes, including fatigue, depression, inhibitions or problems with your partner's technique.
7. This could be caused by fatigue, stress, anxiety or depression—or a hormonal imbalance or clogged arteries.
8. You could have an infection, such as a sexually transmitted disease.
9. This could signal an infection of the prostate gland or urethra.
10. This could be due to an allergy to a contraceptive cream or the rubber in a condom.

Most of these problems are easily treated. While it may seem embarrassing to explain your problem to a doctor, only a doctor can pinpoint the problem and prescribe the treatment necessary.

**Check out hormone replacement therapy.** Researchers have found that postmenopausal women who take testosterone hormones as well as estrogen have enhanced sexual desire and enjoy sex more, says Barbara B. Sherwin, Ph.D., professor in the departments of psychology and obstetrics and gynecology at McGill University and co-director of the McGill University Menopause Clinic at the Jewish General Hospital in Montreal, Quebec. Women who received both hormones "felt better and had more positive moods and greater sexual interest than women treated with estrogen alone," states Dr. Sherwin in *Medical Aspects of Human Sexuality.* (Women naturally produce small amounts of testosterone, and the use of testosterone for reproductive-system problems dates back to the 1940s and 1950s.)

**Cut back on alcohol.** Small amounts of alcohol may stimulate sex drive, but larger amounts or chronic use will depress the desire *and* the ability to perform in both men and women, say experts. Likewise, smoking and drug abuse can put a damper on your sex life.

**Slice the fat from your diet.** A steady diet of cheeseburgers, french fries, cheesecake and other fatty foods may leave you uninterested in sex. Researchers have found that fatty meals may actually curb the production of testosterone, a hormone that can influence sex drive. Four hours after serving fatty shakes to a group of eight men, the researchers saw the men's testosterone levels shrink by nearly a third. When they drank a low-fat beverage of carbohydrates and protein or a nonnutritive drink instead, the sex hormone was unaffected. (Another drawback of fat is that it clogs arteries, including those that rush blood to the penis for an erection.)

# 30

# SLEEP

How to Rest Easy When You Hit the Sack

**Fewer** things restore us more than a good night's sleep. And fewer things are more frustrating than spending a sleepless night tossing and turning—especially when you have a big day ahead of you.

More than 100 million Americans suffer insomnia from time to time, and one out of six has chronic insomnia, spending months or even years troubled by lack of sleep. And insomnia may cause more than daytime sleepiness or fatigue. Eight out of ten people who switch back and forth between day and night shifts have sleep problems, reports the *New England Journal of Medicine,* and they have more heart disease and digestive disorders than people with normal sleep patterns.

### SECRETS OF SOUND SLEEP

Fortunately, researchers have learned much about sleep and how to help people get enough Zs to restore them mentally and physically. After your physician has ruled out any medical cause for your insomnia, give these tips a try.

**Relax!** Sleeping poorly occasionally doesn't interfere too much with your performance the next day, says Peter Hauri, Ph.D., director of the Mayo Clinic Insomnia Program in Rochester, Minnesota. Also, sleep needs vary considerably among people. While the average adult gets about seven hours per night, many people do fine on as few as four to six hours.

**Stick to a schedule.** Even if you've slept poorly the previous night, get up at about the same time you normally do, suggest James K. Walsh, Ph.D., and Mark W. Mahowald, M.D., in an article in *Postgraduate Medicine*. And this means weekends, too! Rising at the same time every day helps maintain a consistent circadian rhythm—the 24-hour internal body clock that keeps us naturally awake during the day and asleep at night. Over time, you'll become sleepy about the same hour each day.

**Limit naps to one hour.** Naps less than an hour may help revitalize you, especially after a restless night. But longer ones will keep you from feeling sleepy at bedtime. Also, sleep *only* in your bed—this includes naps.

**Work out so you can rest easy.** Being inactive can contribute to insomnia. Regular exercise in the late afternoon makes your body temperature rise and then fall as you cool down, and that decrease helps you sleep, say sleep experts. The exercise should be more vigorous than leisurely walking—fast walking, bicycling, jogging and swimming are good—and should be done three to four times a week for at least 20 minutes. Avoid working out within three hours of bedtime, or you could be too revved-up to sleep.

**Watch what you drink—and when.** Alcohol also reduces your amount of deep sleep, so don't drink it within two hours of bedtime, advise Herbert Benson, M.D., and Eileen Stuart, R.N., in *The Wellness Book*. And cut out caffeine by midday: Five to seven hours after you ingest it, half the caffeine is still in your system. (Many foods, beverages and medications contain caffeine, so you'll have to check labels carefully.) Common culprits are coffee products, tea, colas and chocolate or cocoa. Also, if you routinely have to get up at night to urinate, stop drinking liquids after 6:00 P.M.

**Ditch the sleep aids.** If you rely on sleeping pills for more than an occasional bout of insomnia, ask your doctor's advice about how to cut back safely. These drugs decrease the amount of deep, "quality" sleep. So while you may get to sleep sooner, your sleep is poorer. Also, sleeping pills tend to lose their effectiveness after a few weeks of continued use, and they can have a hangover effect the following morning.

**Make the bedroom peaceful.** If you're a light sleeper, you may need to create a kind of "sensory deprivation zone" out of your bedroom. Is there too much light or noise in your bedroom? Is it too warm? Do your cats wake you up with the slightest stirring? Although some people find the hum of a fan, air conditioner or commercially available sound conditioner soothing, others need total silence. And most people sleep best if the room is somewhat cool.

Be sure to use your bedroom only for pleasurable activities—not for anything stressful. Move the computer, desk and other work-related furnishings to the den. You want to associate your bed with relaxation and sleep, not deadlines and household bills.

**Finish the day off.** Plan tomorrow's activities and review the events of the day at least two hours before bedtime. And forget the litany of murder and tragedy on the late news. This is your wind-down period before sleep.

**If you're not sleepy, don't go to bed.** The more time you spend in bed, says Dr. Hauri, the more difficult it can be to fall asleep. Spend no more than six or seven hours in bed. (For most people, this means going to bed an hour or two later than usual.) This will help create a sleep debt, and you'll more likely be ready for sleep when you finally fall into the sack.

**Relax first.** When you get into bed, don't even think about sleeping. Instead, relax for 15 to 20 minutes by reading or listening to music or using relaxation techniques, meditation or prayer. Then turn out the lights to go to sleep. If you're still awake 20 minutes later, leave the room, and don't come back until you feel drowsy again.

## ANTI-AGING CHECKUP
# ARE YOU GETTING ENOUGH SLEEP?

Everyone suffers an occasional restless night. So how can you tell if lack of sleep is not merely an annoyance but a real problem? To help find out, answer the following questions Yes or No.

_____ Is disturbed sleep affecting your mood or job performance?

_____ Do you fall asleep easily at inappropriate moments during the day or while sitting at your desk, the dinner table or a movie?

_____ Do you suffer from daytime sleepiness, lack of energy, tiredness and fatigue?

_____ Do you routinely find it difficult to fall asleep at night?

_____ Do you snore, or are you restless during sleep?

## INTERPRETING YOUR ANSWERS

If the answer is Yes to any of these questions, you'll want to try the tips described in this chapter. But if your wakefulness is caused by arthritis pain, shortness of breath, heartburn, leg cramps, angina or other physical symptoms, see your doctor about these conditions. Also, if your bed partner tells you that you are snoring deeply and having irregular breathing patterns during the night, you may have sleep apnea, which can cause daytime drowsiness, decreased deep sleep and even serious cardiac problems. See your doctor.

# 31

# STOMACH PROBLEMS

## Help for a Sensitive Digestive Tract

You just ate something, and once it hit your stomach, everything was on fire. Yow!

Or you're queasy for no obvious reason. Or something you ate leaves you feeling as though little men are rearranging furniture in your belly.

Or you've got gas.

The medical word for these conditions is *dyspepsia*, but we know it as indigestion. Both words cover a multitude of ailments: nausea, regurgitation (or backwash of stomach contents into the esophagus), vomiting, heartburn, bloating, gas, pain or discomfort, early fullness or whatever you mean by "that sick feeling in my stomach." Whatever the problem, you're wondering why such things happen and, more important, how to get rid of the problem. Here are some answers.

### DIET TIPS FOR A DISTRESS-FREE STOMACH

You may have a sensitive stomach, but it probably isn't a food allergy. "There are very few people who suffer from stomach problems caused by food allergies," says Marvin Schuster, M.D., chief of the division of digestive diseases and professor of medicine at Johns Hopkins University School of Medicine in Baltimore. "Those who do usually have immediate reactions to very specific foods, such as protein foods, lobster or seafood. Often, these people will have hives or abdominal cramps, but there's nothing vague about the reaction. It's immediate, and it can be severe."

Food *intolerances* are more common, says Dr. Schuster, and the most common is lactose intolerance. Here's what to do.

**Monitor your milk.** Every day, radio and TV commercials encourage us to consume milk because it's good for bones, teeth and skin. But many adults can't tolerate milk or milk products because they are unable to digest lactose, the sugar in dairy foods. To do that, you need a particular enzyme called lactase in your intestines—but some people stop producing this enzyme once they're past childhood.

"Lactose intolerance is highly ethnic in its distribution," says Dr. Schuster. "Ninety percent of Chinese are lactose intolerant by the time they reach adolescence. Seventy percent of blacks and 30 to 40 percent of Mediterranean people are as well." *Anyone* can be lactose intolerant, however, no matter what their race or ethnic origin.

Some people are more intolerant than others. "Some people can drink half a cup of milk before they have a reaction; others, only a quarter cup; still others need only a single slice of white bread, which can contain milk, to have a reaction," says Dr. Schuster.

**Make up for missing lactose.** If you don't want to give up dairy foods, you can buy lactase supplements to add to foods to help digest milk products. You can also buy milk with lactase, reduced-lactose cheeses or yogurt with live cultures, which helps to break down the lactose.

**Consume more calcium.** If you do give up milk products, you need to make sure to keep up your calcium intake. Nondairy sources of calcium include foods such as fish canned with bones (salmon, sardines), broccoli, kale and Swiss chard. However, it is difficult to get enough calcium without *any* dairy products, and calcium supplements may be required in individuals who cannot tolerate dairy foods even with lactase supplements.

OTHER THREATS TO AVOID

Be kind to your stomach in other ways by avoiding or cutting back on potential irritants, including these common problem-causers.

**Trim the fat.** "Most people with gastrointestinal problems have some degree of intolerance to fat," says Dr. Schuster. Fat can also contribute to both colon and pancreas cancer by increasing the concentration of bile, says Ronald L. Hoffman, M.D., founder and director of the Hoffman Center for Holistic Medicine in New York.

**Say no to cigarettes.** Smoking elevates the quantity of stomach acids you produce and, at the same time, reduces the natural buffers produced by your pancreas. This is one way smoking promotes ulcers.

**Do without beer, wine and mixed drinks.** Alcohol increases production of gastric acids, while it decreases the amount of pancreatic enzymes used to digest foods. The combination prevents absorption of nutrients, harms digestion and creates digestive disorders. Alcohol also kills friendly bacteria, which assist in digestion.

**Cut out coffee and tea.** Or at least choose decaffeinated versions—and watch out for caffeine-containing sodas as well. Caffeine promotes gastric acid secretion and increases peristalsis, creating a laxative effect. It also interferes with nutrient absorption.

**Don't overdo fiber intake.** Many people do not tolerate wheat, oats or some other grain, says Dr. Schuster. And large amounts of bran can cause problems. "Adding bran to food can cause gas in some people because it ferments in the intestinal tract. A lot of elderly people cannot tolerate a lot of bran," Dr. Schuster says. If you want to add fiber in any form to your diet, do it gradually, preferably in the form of whole foods rather than fiber supplements or bran.

**Check out your water supply.** According to the *American Journal of Public Health*, 35 percent of the gastrointestinal illnesses reported in 606 households studied were related to the tap water they drank. Consider having your water analyzed. The cost of water filters is not exorbitant and may be worth the investment. Or you could buy spring water that is free of harmful bacteria and metals.

**Use aspirin or aspirin alternatives with caution.** Currently, aspirin is hailed as a therapy for heart and circulatory disorders because it promotes circulation by interfering with the blood's tendency to clot. But that same anti-clotting property can promote bleeding in the stomach. "Aspirin can produce gastritis, which is inflammation of the stomach," says Dr. Schuster. "It can also cause bleeding ulcers." Other medications, such as ibuprofen and prescription nonsteroidal anti-inflammatory medicines, have the same negative effect and—like aspirin—should be avoided by anyone with chronic stomach distress.

### Eight Simple, Sensible Stomach Protectors

Once you've eliminated the standard digestive assaults, try eating by the following rules.

**Chew, chew, chew.** "Chewing makes the whole remainder of the digestive process easier, allowing your digestive tract to function as it was designed to function," states Gerard Guillory, M.D., in his book, *IBS: A Doctor's Plan for Chronic Digestive Troubles*. Chewing also allows enzymes in your saliva to mix with your food and start the digestive process, which places less stress on the stomach and small intestine. Finally, chewing your food thoroughly slows down your eating speed, which brings less air into the stomach and results in less intestinal gas.

**Don't overeat.** An obvious problem, but we tend to forget that the faster we eat, the greater our tendency to overeat.

**Avoid hot or cold liquids with meals.** Hot drinks stimulate the colon, says Dr. Guillory, which can cause cramps. Excessive consumption of liquids, especially during a meal, may also cause bloating, gas and irritable bowel syndrome (IBS). Carbonated drinks can cause gas and bloating.

**Try eating small but frequent meals.** Four to six *small* meals a day may be easier for your stomach to take than two or three large ones, says Dr. Guillory.

**Skip the after-dinner mints.** It was widely believed for generations that peppermints aided digestion. However, research demonstrates that peppermints relax the sphincter muscle at the esophagus and cause regurgitation and heartburn, says Dr. Schuster.

**Add ginger.** Freshly grated in tea or used in capsule form, ginger has been shown to settle upset stomachs and keep them settled. The British medical journal *Lancet* reports on one study that compared the effects of ginger and Dramamine (a popular over-the-counter medication for motion-induced nausea) on 36 students, all of whom had motion sickness. These brave volunteers rode blindfolded on a chair that tilted and revolved. The ginger group lasted two minutes longer than the Dramamine group before becoming queasy.

Other studies also document ginger's palliative effects. In a study from Denmark, sailors who were given ginger endured four hours of rough seas better than those who were given a placebo. Another Danish study found that pregnant women with severe nausea from morning sickness found blessed relief in powdered ginger.

**Cut back on fruit juices.** Jeffrey S. Hyams, M.D., professor of pediatrics at the University of Connecticut School of Medicine in Farmington, suggests that people with increased gas, loose stools and diarrhea reduce the amount of fruit juice and sugars in their diet. Sugar is sometimes only partially absorbed by the intestinal tract, and leftover sugars are consumed by bacteria, which ferment them and produce hydrogen that can cause gas, bloating and cramps.

**Revamp your diet.** Modern physicians urge us to return to the diet of our ancestors—whole grains, vegetables and fruit—to promote peace and harmony in our digestive tract. "The 'ideal diet' should be high in complex carbohydrates, low in fats (particularly saturated fats and cholesterol), with moderate amounts of protein," says Dr. Guillory. Salt is unrelated, except that it tends to come in high-fat foods, such as fast foods.

**ANTI-AGING CHECKUP**
# DIAGNOSING A TROUBLED STOMACH

Have a chronic stomach problem? Here are the most common causes; check off those that are part of your lifestyle.

\_\_\_\_ Overeating
\_\_\_\_ Caffeine
\_\_\_\_ Alcohol
\_\_\_\_ Tobacco
\_\_\_\_ Fat in the diet
\_\_\_\_ Spicy foods
\_\_\_\_ Eating large meals at night or before lying down

## INTERPRETING YOUR ANSWERS

If you and your physician have ruled out these causes for your tummy troubles, your physician may suggest a special breath test that can be used to determine if you have an intolerance to sugars or some other carbohydrate. The test detects small amounts of hydrogen given off by bacteria that are fermenting undigested carbohydrates. Consequently, it is very accurate, painless and easy to perform. The test is expensive, however, so it will probably be recommended only as a last resort.

# 32

# STRENGTH

### Easy Weight Training for Better Bodies

**Strong,** healthy muscle is the foundation of physical beauty. And that's not Madison Avenue talking; it's the implicit message of Michelangelo and Leonardo da Vinci as well as all the Greek sculptors. Strong and healthy muscle is part of what makes the human body a noble and wondrous work of art.

But stronger muscles can do more than just make you *look* good. Strength training will not only consume calories but also speed metabolism and help weight loss. It can also restore range of motion to people suffering from arthritis, allowing them to return to recreational and work-related activities.

When we exercise, our nerves and muscles become better coordinated to make performance more efficient and graceful. Despite these benefits, anyone with high blood pressure, heart disease or any other serious medical condition should consult their physician before starting any kind of weight-training program.

The benefits of healthy muscle go far beyond physical beauty, however. Well-conditioned muscles also:

- store greater amounts of energy that's there when you need it. Muscles act like warehouses of energy, and the stronger and larger the muscle, the greater the available energy.
- improve strength and endurance, allowing us to work harder and longer without experiencing fatigue or weakness.

- provide greater mobility and independence well into old age. In this way, the loss of function associated with aging is slowed.
- strengthen bones, prevent bone loss due to osteoporosis and reduce the likelihood of fractures.
- protect us from injury by cushioning falls better than muscle-deficient or fatty tissues.
- protect against low-back pain and injury, often caused by weakened muscles in the abdomen, lower back and kidney area.
- improve virtually all aspects of life, from the simple chores of lifting groceries to meeting life's challenges at work and play.

## WEIGHT-TRAINING OPTIONS

Anyone considering resistance training can choose from a variety of weights, materials and configurations. Free weights can be small, hand-held dumbbells, ankle or wrist weights of 1 to 10 pounds or heavier barbells. However, barbell training should be supervised, especially if you are new to weight training, warns Roger Fielding, exercise physiologist at the U.S. Department of Agriculture's Human Nutrition Research Center on Aging at Tufts University in Boston.

Hand and wrist weights are generally inexpensive, but you can bypass the cost entirely by filling empty bleach bottles with water or sand. The handles make lifting easier to manage, so the weights are less likely to fall on your feet.

"You can also use rubber exercise bands," says Fielding. "The problem with exercise bands, however, is that you cannot easily increase the resistance as you can with weights. If you're working with only one or two bands, you will not be able to extend your strength beyond those resistances."

YMCAs and private and university health and fitness clubs offer a full line of weight and exercise equipment you can use at surprisingly little cost. Ask personnel to demonstrate the machines for you.

## GET OFF TO A GOOD START

So you've found a gym or bought some equipment—or made your own—and you're ready to start your strength-training program. These tips will help ensure the success of your program.

**Dress comfortably.** You don't need to buy special attire, but choose comfortable clothing. Sweat suits and sneakers are fine.

**Warm up first.** Do some walking or light jogging, even in place, to prepare the body for exercise.

**Find a partner.** If at all possible, exercise with a partner who can assist you if you have trouble with your weights. If you are an older person and new to weight training, do the exercises while sitting or holding on to a chair that's firm and stable.

**Remember to breathe.** Exhale as you lift, and inhale while you lower the weights. Breathe evenly throughout the exercise. Do not hold your breath at any point. That can raise your blood pressure considerably.

**Support your back.** When lifting from a seated position, be sure to place your lower back against the chair.

**Allow a rest.** Rest two minutes between sets or until you feel ready to continue.

**Start with your legs.** Exercise the large muscle groups in your legs first, before moving on to the arms and abdomen. This will increase circulation, which will improve your endurance and allow you to exercise longer before tiring.

**Stop if you're in pain.** If you feel any pain, stop the exercise. A mild burning sensation is normal with resistance efforts, but any acute or stabbing pain is a warning that you are straining too hard or performing the maneuver incorrectly.

## PLANNING YOUR WORKOUT

You can develop your own workout program, do the exercises listed here or ask a health-club professional or physical therapist to design a program for you.

It's best to start with light weights—a pound or two—for the first week, especially if this is the first time you've tried strength training. If that feels comfortable, increase the weights the next week, and so on.

After you're comfortable with the weights and want to get stronger, you should use a weight that is at least 70 percent of the maximum you can lift. "We recommend 3 sets, each made up of 8 to 10 repetitions of an exercise," says Fielding. "We also recommend that you do these sets three to four times a week. After seven or eight weeks, you will have reached a level of conditioning at which you'll only have to do the training twice a week to maintain strength and fitness."

As you improve, you'll need to increase the weight so that you're still lifting 70 percent of your maximum. At some point, you'll want to level off and stay with the same weight. This will keep up your current level of strength and fitness but won't make you any stronger.

### A Sample Program

A good range of exercises includes the following moves.

**Extend your lower legs.** Using ankle weights, sit on a sturdy desk or a high chair, with your legs dangling. Lift one leg straight out so it is nearly parallel to the floor. Hold for 1 count, then slowly lower the leg completely. Do 8 to 10 repetitions, alternating legs.

**Curl your hamstrings.** To do this exercise, you'll need ankle weights. Support yourself by holding on to the back of a chair. While balancing on one leg, raise the ankle of the other leg toward the buttocks. Slowly lower your foot to the floor. Do 8 to 10 repetitions, alternating legs.

**Do calf lifts.** Place the balls of your feet on a thick book, while supporting yourself by holding on to the back of a chair or table. Raise your body by going up on your tiptoes, then slowly lower yourself until your heels are just below the level of the book and your Achilles tendons are stretching somewhat. Repeat 8 to 10 times.

**Develop your bench press.** You can do this from the floor with hand weights or from a specially designed bench with a barbell. Lift the weights from your chest directly upward until your elbows are only slightly bent, while exhaling. Lower them slowly while extending your arms outward in a semicircle, inhaling. Do 8 to 10 repetitions.

**Perform arm curls.** Holding a barbell or hand weights, curl the weight toward your chest while sitting, supporting your lower back against the back of the chair. Do 8 to 10 repetitions.

**Curl the wrists, too.** Rest your forearm on a table with your hand over the edge, palm up. Place a weight in your hand, and lift it toward you as far as you can—without lifting your forearm off the table—then slowly return it to a resting position. Do 8 to 10 repetitions, alternating hands.

**Sit up—the new way.** Lie on the floor and bend your knees, with your lower back pressed into the floor. Either cross your arms over your chest or place your fingers lightly behind your ears. Raise your upper back a few inches off the floor, then slowly lower yourself back down, without letting your head quite touch the floor. (Don't, however, use your arms to swing your body forward. You want your stomach muscles to do the work—not your back.) Do 8 to 10 repetitions. This type of sit-up is called a crunch.

### LOWER THE WEIGHT WITH CARE

Weight and resistance training strengthens muscles by breaking down old proteins, which are then replaced by larger and stronger muscle fibers. Weight training has two phases: lifting the weight and lowering it. Actually, lowering weights—working with gravity—does the most to make muscles grow. Raising weights is essential, of course, but it doesn't have quite as much muscle-enlarging effect as lowering. "We recommend that you lift the weights, hold them at their peak for a second, and then allow them to descend slowly over three seconds," says Fielding. That ensures that the descent—or what trainers call the eccentric phase of the exercise—does you the most good.

### INTERIOR BODY BUILDING

As mentioned earlier, muscles become stronger by breaking down protein fibers. Contrary to a longstanding myth, nutritionists do not recommend that people increase their protein intake to accommodate a weight-training program. In a normal diet, we get all the protein we need to build strong muscles. (Anyone who is malnourished or on a very restricted diet, however, may not have sufficient intake of energy or protein to support muscle growth during resistance training.) If you add more protein to your diet, it will likely be eliminated from the body. Most of us need to eat more complex carbohydrates, found in whole grains, breads, vegetables and fruits, which provide abundant sources of energy. You'll likely have a more comfortable workout if you eat only lightly before a strength-training session, however.

---

### ANTI-AGING CHECKUP
## HOW MUCH SHOULD YOU LIFT?

The ideal weight to train at is somewhere between 70 and 80 percent of the maximum weight that you can bench press or curl. So if your maximum bench press or curl is 50 pounds, you want to train at 35 to 40 pounds. That will ensure that you improve your strength.

However, it's easy to injure yourself while trying to find your maximum. Tufts University researchers recommend that you train with the maximum weight that you can bench press or curl eight to ten times. That weight will be approximately 70 to 80 percent of your maximum.

*Editors note:* Talk to your doctor or physical therapist before starting a weight-training program. This advice is particularly important if your doctor has said you may be at risk for osteoporosis or other health conditions.

# 33

# STROKE

Best Ways to Stack the Cards
in Your Favor

**Every** year, millions of Americans 65 and over—the age-group at high risk for stroke—pack up, bounce out of the house and jump into the car, off for a long vacation or to move to a new locale. They're cashing in on their dreams of the good life.

Why are these older folks healthy and up for adventure? Luck could play a role, but chances are that these "fortunate" folks have been helping their luck along by leading a healthy life. You can share in the same good fortune by making wise lifestyle choices, which can mean the difference between having a healthy, active future and becoming a stroke statistic.

And the statistics are grim. Each year, more than 500,000 Americans suffer a stroke. A third of these are fatal and another third are disabling (some paralysis, memory loss or loss of one or more senses), while the rest suffer no lasting effect.

The most common cause is atherosclerosis, cholesterol plaques that clog the arteries leading to the brain. Often, these plaques cause clots to form in the arteries. Clots can break free of the plaque, travel down the vessel and eventually block the flow of blood and oxygen to the brain. The result is that part of the brain suffocates and dies. Other times, a stroke is caused by a cerebral hemorrhage—a burst blood vessel that floods delicate brain tissue.

#### AGING IS NOT A REQUIREMENT

Stroke is the third-leading killer in the United States, and while it is primarily associated with advancing age, many young people—particularly young women—suffer strokes because they pile up risk factors that lead to the deadly disease. Those who suffer premature strokes fit a certain profile. They:

- use birth control pills.
- have high blood pressure.
- smoke cigarettes.
- abuse drugs and consume too much alcohol.
- have a disorder of the heart's mitral valve.
- have a history of migraine headaches.

"When you think about these risk factors, especially the three main ones—use of oral contraceptives, mild hypertension and smoking—you realize that they're not all that uncommon a cluster," says Michael Weber, M.D., professor of medicine at the University of California, Irvine, College of Medicine. "Together, these do cause strokes in young women." And unlike other segments of the population, young women are smoking *more*, not less, Dr. Weber points out.

One early warning sign of a stroke is the transient ischemic attack (TIA), or ministroke. TIAs temporarily leave the face or limbs numb, impair speech or vision (especially in one eye) or cause periods of weakness or dizziness. The symptoms often pass in less than 24 hours, but ministrokes are a sign that the brain is not getting enough oxygen, and a bigger stroke may be on the way. If at any time you think you are suffering a TIA, get to a doctor fast. Thirty percent of those who experience a TIA go on to have a major stroke, sometimes within weeks or days.

#### STOP A STROKE BEFORE IT STOPS YOU

For many people, lifestyle changes alone are sufficient to reduce the likelihood of stroke, so come out swinging. Don't wait for danger signals; start doing what you can to disarm the enemy.

**Get the drop on blood pressure.** "The first thing you should do to reduce your risk of stroke is lower your blood pressure," says Dr. Weber. You can do this through diet, exercise and—when necessary—medication. As blood pressure drops, so does the risk of stroke—often dramatically.

Among the best ways to lower blood pressure: Lose weight, get regular aerobic exercise and eliminate excess salt from the diet. Salt is a contributor to hypertension in about half of those who suffer from the disease. (See chapter 6.)

**Drop both pounds and cigarettes.** Smoking itself is a major risk factor in the onset of stroke; when it is combined with excess weight, the likelihood of a stroke skyrockets, according to a report in the British medical journal *Lancet*. One study estimated that together, the two account for 60 percent of strokes in men 65 and under.

**Lower those lipids.** A high-fat, high-cholesterol diet raises LDL cholesterol, the type that causes atherosclerosis and contributes to stroke. People with diabetes run a particularly high risk of having a stroke because they often have high blood pressure and high cholesterol levels.

By eating a diet low in fat and cholesterol and rich in grains and vegetables, you prevent stroke in several ways by helping decrease your blood cholesterol and increasing your intake of disease-fighting nutrients. Research shows that people who suffer a stroke generally have lower dietary levels of potassium, calcium and vitamin D than healthy individuals. In one study, healthy women's diets contained 38 percent more vitamin D and 17 percent more calcium than the diets of women who had suffered a stroke.

Studies also show that vitamin E prevents blood platelets from sticking to the walls of arteries and forming cholesterol plaques, a precursor for stroke and other cardiovascular diseases.

When you choose a healthy, low-fat diet, you'll be eating whole grains and seeds rich in vitamin E and leafy greens rich in calcium, plus some of the vegetables and fruits that are good sources of potassium. These anti-stroke foods are also associated with lower blood pressure and blood cholesterol.

## Walk Your Way Out of Danger

Regular aerobic exercise, especially moderate walking, is one of the best ways to prevent stroke, according to the *British Medical Journal*. Researchers examined the exercise and stroke rates of 7,735 men, ages 40 to 59, and concluded that moderate physical activity such as walking significantly reduces the risk of stroke and heart attacks in men, both with and without preexisting heart conditions.

The reason is amazingly simple. Clots are the principal cause of strokes, and exercise increases the clot-dissolving factors in the blood, says Wayne Chandler, M.D., assistant professor of laboratory medicine at the University of Washington in Seattle.

"When exercised, the body produces tissue-plasminogen activator (t-PA), which prevents clots from forming and dissolves existing clots," says Dr. Chandler. Regular moderate exercise, such as walking four or five times a week for 30 minutes, will increase the body's production of t-PA.

Exercise also cuts down on the body's production of the protein fibrinogen, which clots are made of. "Studies suggest that your risk of stroke and heart disease goes up if your fibrinogen levels are higher than normal," says Dr. Chandler. "This combination of decreasing fibrinogen and increasing t-PA may help increase the rate at which you dissolve clots as they start to form."

## Aspirin: Not Just a Headache Remedy

Small doses of aspirin may help prevent a stroke, especially if you have already suffered a TIA or a major stroke. Aspirin reduces the ability of blood platelets to form the clots that clog arteries, cut blood flow and invite stroke.

"For those who have already had vascular disease, either heart attack, angina, stroke or TIA, there is conclusive evidence that low-dose aspirin decreases the risk of subsequent stroke, heart attack or death," says Charles Henneken, M.D., acting chairman of preventive medicine at Harvard Medical School.

Swedish researchers found that a group that took 73 milligrams of aspirin daily (about the amount in a baby aspirin) were 18 percent less likely to have a stroke (or die from one) than those who didn't get aspirin. Also, those who took aspirin were 16 to 20 percent less likely to have a second stroke or heart attack.

A Dutch study shows that 30 milligrams of aspirin daily is as effective at lowering the risk of heart attacks and stroke as a dose commonly used, nearly ten times larger (283 milligrams). (An adult aspirin contains about 325 milligrams.) The lesser amount also results in fewer bleeding complications.

Physicians point out, however, that there may be little or no benefit to taking aspirin to prevent a first stroke. Moreover, some evidence suggests that those who take aspirin to prevent a first heart attack may slightly increase their risk of suffering a stroke.

The bottom line is that you should not take aspirin to protect your heart without first consulting your doctor. Also, the dose prescribed should not be changed—either increased or decreased—without his or her okay.

## ANTI-AGING CHECKUP
# ARE YOU AT RISK FOR A STROKE?

The best indicator of whether you're prone to a stroke is your blood pressure. "Any blood pressure above 95 (diastolic) at the bottom and 140 (systolic) on the top is above normal and should be a concern," says Michael Weber, M.D., professor of medicine at the University of California, Irvine, College of Medicine. "If the person suffers from other risk factors as well, he may be predisposing himself to a stroke."

Are you at risk? Answer the following questions Yes or No.

_____ 1. Do you have high blood pressure?

_____ 2. Do you have heart disease?

_____ 3. Do you smoke?

_____ 4. Do you have a high red blood cell count?

_____ 5. Have you suffered transient ischemic attacks or mini-strokes?

_____ 6. Are you 65 or over? (Only one in seven people who die of stroke is under 65.)

_____ 7. Are you a man? (Men are more prone to strokes than women.)

_____ 8. Do you have diabetes mellitus? (People with diabetes have a higher incidence of stroke.)

_____ 9. Have you had a stroke before?

_____ 10. Do you have a family history of stroke?

_____ 11. Do you have an asymptomatic carotid bruit? (This is a carotid artery involvement or blockage disclosed by stethoscope sound detected by a physician.)

_____ 12. Are you African-American? (Blacks are more prone to stroke than whites.)

_____ 13. Do you have atrial fibrillation?

_____ 14. Do you have a high cholesterol level?

If you answered question 1 Yes and gave a Yes answer to any other question, you may be at risk for a stroke. The more Yes answers you have, the higher your chances of stroke, and the more important it is that you take action to prevent a problem. If you had more than one Yes answer—or didn't know the answer to a question—check with your doctor.

# 34

# TASTE AND SMELL

Your Link to Some of Life's
Finest Pleasures

**What** would food be without our sense of taste? What about the pleasures we'd miss from flowers or a pine forest if we had no sense of smell? It's easy to take those senses for granted—until they become impaired.

It's taste and smell that make life intimate. And these senses stimulate memory as well. It's natural to associate specific smells and tastes with events in our lives. When we reencounter these sensations—the scent of a lover's perfume, a sip of a wine first tasted in an exotic locale—they may release a flood of feelings or memories that cause a delectable déjà vu.

## Senses That Would Be Sorely Missed

Taste and smell can alert us to danger—the smell of smoke or poisonous fumes, the taste of spoiled food or ingredients we are allergic to. And when the ability to taste or smell is impaired, we may be unable to make appropriate food choices. This can cause poor dietary habits that lead to illness, loss of appetite, weight loss and deficiencies in certain nutrients, such as calcium and vitamins A and C. Those with a diminished sense of taste or smell often try to compensate by adding excessive amounts of flavor enhancers—such as sugar and salt—to foods. Others overeat simply because they don't feel satisfied after eating what they didn't taste.

Experts estimate that nearly two million Americans suffer

from lost or distorted taste and smell. Such impairment can strike people of any age, but it happens most often from ages 65 to 80.

What dulls these senses? Taste and smell are delicate and mutually dependent. The tongue can discern only four distinct tastes—sweet, salty, sour and bitter. We can distinguish so many more flavors and nuances of flavor because much of what we perceive as taste is actually smell.

We all recognize this interdependency whenever we suffer from a head cold. A stuffed nose reduces our sense of taste to a fraction of its normal sharpness. In fact, upper-respiratory disorders—nasal and sinus trouble or lung infections—are the most common reasons people suffer a temporary diminished capacity for taste.

## RECULTIVATE YOUR SENSE OF TASTE AND SMELL

Most loss of taste is actually due to problems with the sense of smell. These include injury to olfactory nerves because of exposure to toxic chemicals, head injury, surgery involving the face or skull, certain types of seizure disorders, stroke, endocrine gland malfunction and birth defects.

Though less common than damage to the smell apparatus, disorders that affect the sense of taste alone do exist. Among these are degeneration of the oral cavity, dry mouth (xerostomia), radiation therapy, certain viral infections, endocrine gland disorders and direct injury.

If you have experienced a loss of taste or smell, check with your doctor to determine the cause. And these three tips may help restore those senses.

**Kick the habit.** Cigarette smoking is a common cause of impaired taste and smell. A study conducted by University of Pennsylvania researchers shows that people who smoke are twice as likely to have a diminished sense of taste and smell than nonsmokers. Other studies show that cigarette smoking changes olfactory nerve tissue in mice and progressively reduces their ability to smell.

These senses do return when the smoking stops! But don't expect your powers of taste and smell to kick in again the day or even weeks after you swear off cigarettes. Still, the sooner you stop, the sooner you'll regain the power of these senses.

**Think about zinc.** A widely used medical treatment for losses of smell and taste—and one of the most successful—is a zinc sulfate supplement. This helps restore taste and smell acuity in people with kidney and liver diseases that affect blood levels of zinc. If you have such a condition, ask your doctor if zinc is worth a try.

**Train your nose.** Scientists at Monell Chemical Senses Center in Philadelphia found that people who are "smell-blind" to a particular fragrance or odor can develop the ability to recognize that smell after continued exposure to it. In one case, the scientists exposed a group of people to a chemical substance called androstenone, which the people initially could not smell. During the study, half of those who had been smell-blind to androstenone became able to recognize its odor.

### DRY MOUTH MUFFLES FLAVOR

Food must dissolve on taste buds so you can taste it. But that process is hampered in the millions of Americans who suffer from dry mouth syndrome, xerostomia.

How do you get such an ailment in the first place? Between 250 and 300 common medications can cause dry mouth syndrome, including many diuretics, blood pressure drugs, antihistamines and antidepressants. Even caffeinated beverages have been shown to cause xerostomia. However, several effective methods of relief are readily available. These are among the most commonly recommended.

**Reach for a lemon drop.** Citric acid stimulates saliva, so lemon drops can moisten your mouth, say experts. Also, sugarless mints can produce a tenfold increase in saliva production, according to a study at Columbia University's Center for Clinical Research in Dentistry. Chewing sugarless gum and sucking on other sugarless candies also increases saliva.

**Drown the drys.** Are you drinking enough? Stick to non-caffeinated beverages because caffeine is a diuretic and may contribute to dry mouth.

**Try artificial saliva.** Sprayed into the mouth, artificial saliva medication can be prescribed by physicians. Ask your doctor about it.

**Review your diet.** Keep track of what you eat and drink, and try to determine the food or beverage that causes the dry mouth. Eliminate that particular item to see if your symptoms disappear.

---

### ANTI-AGING CHECKUP
# HOW WELL DO YOU SMELL AND TASTE?

It's fun and easy to test your senses of smell and taste. You'll probably find what's needed for this at-home checkup, well, right at home.

### SMELL TESTER

Gather the following:

- perfume or fresh flowers
- onion or garlic
- chocolate
- mint
- instant coffee
- turpentine
- fresh tobacco (preferably pipe tobacco)
- a snuffed-out paper match

Have someone select any three items from the list and place them—one at a time—under your nose while your eyes are closed. Then try to identify the smell of each.

### TASTE TESTER

There are four basic tastes—sweet, salty, sour and bitter. Taste buds that perceive sweet taste are located at the tip of the tongue; salty, on the top of the tongue toward the front; sour, along the sides of the tongue; bitter, at the back. To test how

*continued*

well you detect each one of them, prepare the following mixtures.

- Salty: one teaspoon of salt dissolved in four ounces of distilled water
- Sour: one teaspoon of vinegar dissolved in one ounce of distilled water
- Sweet: one teaspoon of sugar dissolved in four ounces of distilled water
- Bitter: quinine water (tonic water)

Place a drop of each on the part of the tongue where the flavor's corresponding taste buds are located. Put a drop of sweet water on the tip of the tongue, a drop of bitter at the back, and so on. Your sensory response to this test will tell you how well your power of taste is functioning.

# 35

# ULCERS

New Thinking about Causes and Cures

**The** classic symptom is all too familiar: a gnawing stomach pain that usually occurs at night or a few hours after a meal. While this can suggest a number of different problems, it may also point to a stomach ulcer.

Ten percent of Americans will develop a stomach ulcer sometime in their lives. Though we frequently associate ulcers with job stress, experts agree that your lifestyle and the types of medications you take have much more to do with these stomach sores.

The truth is, most people who suffer from ulcers actually contribute to the disorder themselves—which means they can help heal it, too. With proper treatment, ulcers can be cured, usually within 12 weeks.

## How Ulcers Are Created

Stomach ulcers are craterlike sores that develop either in the lining of the stomach (gastric ulcers) or in the duodenum, the first stage of the small intestine (duodenal ulcers). An ulcer can range from tiny sores to major areas of corrosion one-fourth inch to two inches in diameter.

The stomach itself is a muscular sac that churns food and digestive juices into an emulsified mix that's sent on to the small intestine, where the nutrients are absorbed. The two primary stomach juices involved are hydrochloric acid and pepsin.

The lining of the stomach is a mucous membrane that, if damaged, can expose underlying sensitive tissues to these powerful digestive secretions. These compounds can eat away part of the exposed tissue, causing a sore or ulcer. Sometimes the sore develops first, due to bacteria or drugs, and is then exposed to the hydrochloric acid and pepsin. In either case, the stomach actually breaks down its own tissues and digests them.

A gastric ulcer can grow deep enough to pierce the lining of the stomach and cause internal bleeding. An untreated duodenal ulcer can become so big that it blocks food from passing from the stomach to the small intestine. This usually results in vomiting of food and blood.

Both gastric and duodenal ulcers can be life-threatening, so immediate medical attention is critical—and, luckily, effective. Ninety to 95 percent of all ulcers are treated successfully, *without* surgery.

## DON'T BLAME SPICY FOODS

Many people think that hot, spicy foods are a major cause of ulcers, but scientists have not proved that, says Marvin Schuster, M.D., chief of the division of digestive diseases and professor of medicine at Johns Hopkins University School of Medicine in Baltimore. Truth be told, the common causes of ulcers are:

- cigarette smoking;
- overuse of nonsteroidal anti-inflammatory drugs (NSAIDs) such as aspirin or ibuprofen;
- infection of the stomach by a type of bacteria.

Stress, alcohol and other lifestyle and dietary factors may play a role, but scientists are less certain of just how much damage they do.

### ULCER-FIGHTING STRATEGIES

There are plenty of weapons in the battle against ulcers. Here are some ways to help quiet these sores or lessen your chances of getting them.

**If you smoke, quit.** "Smoking doubles your chances of getting an ulcer," states an article in the *Johns Hopkins Medical Letter*. "It will also slow the healing of ulcers and make them likely to recur."

Scientists are not entirely sure how smoking causes ulcers. The stomach, like all tissue, is continually healing itself from a variety of insults, says Naurang Agrawal, M.D., a gastroenterologist at the Ochsner Clinic in New Orleans. But smoking interrupts this healing process, thus predisposing the smoker to ulcers. The bottom line: Add ulcers to the list of trouble caused by smoking.

**Ditch the NSAIDs.** Nonsteroidal anti-inflammatory drugs which you may take to treat aches, pains or inflammation, include aspirin, ibuprofen (a major ingredient in Motrin, Advil and Nuprin) and some prescription drugs. All are known to injure the stomach's protective mucous lining and thereby expose the tissues to acid and pepsin. If you have an ulcer, reach for acetaminophen for minor ailments. If your doctor has prescribed an NSAID, ask if another medication can be substituted.

**Ask about an NSAID antidote.** People with arthritis and other illnesses associated with inflammation sometimes must continue to take NSAIDs. Misoprostol, a synthetic prostaglandin, significantly reduces the incidence of gastric ulcers in people who take NSAIDs. In one study, reported in the *Annals of Internal Medicine*, only 2 people of 122 involved developed stomach ulcers after taking both misoprostol and NSAIDs. In a control group of 131 people taking only NSAIDs, 21 people got stomach ulcers.

**Battle bacteria with antibiotics.** *Helicobacter pylori,* a common bacteria, can take up residence in the stomach and have a corrosive effect on the lining similar to that of NSAIDs. Not everyone infected with this bacteria gets ulcers, however. "There are more people with *H. pylori* who do not have ulcers than those who have the bacteria and get ulcers," says Dr. Agrawal. Why the bacteria causes ulcers in some and not all is still a mystery. Fortunately, antibiotics can wipe out the bacteria, and studies show that when *H. pylori* is eradicated, stomach ulcers heal.

**Consider the stress factor.** Today's world makes stress as much a guarantee as death and taxes. And most of us believe that stress at least contributes to ulcers, if it doesn't actually cause them, although science hasn't confirmed that theory.

Emotional responses—including stress—are difficult to measure. Also, each of us tends to see situations in a different way: What's stressful for one might not be stressful for another. But a study published in the *Archives of Internal Medicine* that followed 4,511 people over an eight-year period found that those who perceived themselves as stressed were nearly twice as likely to suffer ulcers as people who felt stress-free. There are many effective ways to deal with stress, including positive imaging routines, prayer, meditation and exercise. (See chapter 59.)

**Booze does not soothe.** People often respond to stress by having a few beers, a couple of glasses of wine or another form of alcohol. But drinking tends to elevate acid production in the stomach. Alcohol-induced cirrhosis of the liver is associated with increased risk of ulcers. And drinking, like smoking, prevents the stomach from healing. Still, the question of whether alcohol causes this itself or acts with other factors, such as stress, remains unanswered. In any case, if you have an ulcer, the best thing to do is eliminate alcohol to let your stomach heal.

**Broccoli beats buttercreams.** Despite numerous studies, a correlation between high fiber intake and a lower incidence of duodenal ulcers has yet to be proven. A British study published in the medical journal *Gut* showed a strong connection between refined sugar intake and ulcers. It made a smaller, but still significant, association between a higher vegetable-fiber intake and a lower incidence of duodenal ulcers.

Other research shows that sugar increases fermentation and stimulates intestinal bacteria to produce hydrogen gas. The hydrogen causes an array of stomach problems, including gas, bloating, distention and cramps.

While researchers continue to examine and haggle over unresolved questions, it's wise for people with ulcers to increase their intake of vegetables and reduce or eliminate refined sugars.

**Don't reach for the moo-juice.** Despite evidence to the contrary, some still believe the myth that milk is good for stomach ulcers. Years ago, doctors seemed to think that milk protectively coats the stomach, much the way it coats the inside of a glass. But scientists have since discovered that the calcium and protein in milk actually stimulate increased production of hydrochloric acids and other digestive juices, which literally attack an ulcer. Those with sensitive stomachs are better off avoiding milk.

## Be Alert for Side Effects

If these self-help measures aren't effective or if your ulcers are severe, your doctor may prescribe a medication such as Tagamet. But a possible side effect of these drugs, called H2 receptor blockers, is breast enlargement and breast sensitivity in both men and women, says Dr. Schuster. If you experience either of these symptoms, consult your physician and ask about alternatives.

Also, the long-term use of ulcer-fighting products that block the secretion of acid can interfere with your absorption of essential nutrients, including iron, calcium, folate and vitamin $B_{12}$. So experts caution that you take these drugs no longer than necessary.

You should also take care if you're reaching for an antacid for relief. Scientists warn that such medications, while usually providing immediate relief, may increase the incidence of diarrhea and the risk of contracting kidney disease. Antacids that result in the fewest side effects are DiGel, Maalox, Mylanta and Riopan, say the editors of the *Johns Hopkins Health Letter*. If you habitually take antacids for stomach distress, consult your doctor about another approach.

**ANTI-AGING CHECKUP**
# SO, YOU THINK YOU'RE GETTING AN ULCER . . .

Answer Yes or No to these questions to determine if you have symptoms of an ulcer.

____ Do you have chronic pain in the stomach? The pain can be sharp or dull and may radiate from the stomach to the back.

____ Do you suffer from chronic nausea or regurgitation of acid or partially digested food into the mouth?

____ Do you experience a gradual or sudden onset of weakness, dizziness or pale skin?

____ Are you vomiting blood or a substance that looks like coffee grounds?

____ Have your stools changed color to dark black or maroon?

## INTERPRETING YOUR ANSWERS

If any of these problems occur, see your physician immediately.

# 36

# VARICOSE VEINS

Gnarly Legs *Aren't* Inevitable

**Varicose** veins can make your legs look like colorful road maps. In many cases, they even take on topographical features, mounds and bumps that rise above the surface of the skin.

Veins carry blood filled with carbon dioxide back to the heart and lungs. Like salmon swimming upstream, the blood in your legs must defy gravity to get back to the heart. The muscles in your legs contract with every step you take, helping pump the blood upward.

Inside the veins are valves, much like trapdoors, that keep the blood from flowing backward. Under certain conditions, the vein may swell, preventing the valve from closing properly, or the valve itself may weaken and leak. In either case, blood gets trapped inside the vein, where it collects and causes the vein to bulge. Smaller expansions, called spider veins, can appear on the legs, ankles and face and can be red, blue or purple, and they're usually painless. (See chapter 47.)

Varicose veins are larger vessels near the surface of the skin that have ballooned and become permanently swollen with blood and are usually blue or purple. Besides being unpleasant to look at, they can cause a variety of problems, such as throbbing, heaviness, night cramps and long-term complications such as ulcerations and bleeding.

Most people who suffer from varicose veins deal with the problem by covering their legs with long dresses, pants or thick hose. But that's a stopgap measure, not a solution. There are answers. Varicose veins can be prevented and successfully treated.

## A Family Heritage You Can Do Without

"Varicose veins run in families, much like baldness," says Walter De Groot, M.D., president of the North American Society of Phlebology in Seattle. Gender is also a factor: Half of American women over the age of 40, but only 10 percent of men, suffer from varicose veins. The reason for the contrasting incidence lies in hormonal differences between the sexes and in pregnancy.

Pregnancy predisposes women to varicose veins in two ways: The growing baby puts pressure on the circulation in the legs and lower part of the body. Also, the level of estrogen in a woman's body rises during pregnancy, causing the muscles in the walls of all the vessels to relax and virtually encouraging them to bulge.

While these conditions set the stage for varicose veins, that doesn't mean they are inevitable, as many people—some doctors included—believe. One surgeon writing in a popular magazine once described varicose veins as "the price the human race pays for walking upright." But that isn't true. Researchers have established that the disorder is rare in Third World countries. The *Southern Medical Journal* carried a report by researchers Glenn W. Geelhoed, M.D., and Denis P. Burkitt, M.D., stating that "varicose veins are nonexistent to rare in whole populations of the developing world."

Unfortunately, when members of these low-risk populations, such as those in Africa or Asia, come to the West and adopt Western diets and lifestyles, their rates of varicose veins shoot upward. For example, while the problem is uncommon among Africans, their African-American counterparts suffer from varicose veins as much as white Americans do.

## Raise Your Self-Defense Quotient

Dr. Geelhoed and Dr. Burkitt say that lifestyle factors—especially diet and exercise—play a far more important role than is currently recognized. They believe that varicose veins may well be preventable, and many of their colleagues agree. Here are some of the ways you can keep your veins from bulging as well as help prevent mild venous problems from getting worse.

**Vitamins C and E offer vessel insurance.** Studies show that vitamins C and E—both antioxidants, which help stabilize and heal tissues—may help maintain elasticity of blood vessels, says Conrad Goulet, M.D., owner of Guylaine Lanctot Institute in Palm Beach Gardens, Florida, a clinic that specializes in the treatment of varicose veins. Eat foods rich in C and E, such as citrus fruits, especially if varicose veins run in your family, he recommends.

**Fiber and digestion play a part, too.** A high-fiber diet may lower the risk of varicose veins by making bowel movements less strenuous. Low-fiber diets, on the other hand, result in greater straining during bowel evacuation. That pressure is transmitted down the legs and impacts directly against the valves in the veins. Dr. Geelhoed and Dr. Burkitt point out that Western populations that eat low-fiber diets pass smaller and firmer stools than do less industrialized populations that have low rates of varicose veins.

**Eat a low-fat diet.** Fat is known to cause heart and vascular diseases, which, according to Dr. Geelhoed and Dr. Burkitt, may be related to the onset of varicose veins. The researchers urge people to adopt a diet rich in grains, vegetables, fruit and fiber—a reflection of the primitive diet that they call the Paleolithic prescription—as a means of avoiding multiple illnesses as well as preventing varicose veins.

**Lose excess weight.** Obesity can contribute to several circulatory disorders, including high blood pressure. Increased blood pressure may damage valves, causing swelling or leaks. Excess fat on the legs increases the difficulty of pumping blood upward and back to the heart.

**Stop smoking.** The Framingham Heart Study, a long-term study gathering health-related data on the adult residents of Framingham, Massachusetts, shows a correlation between smoking and the incidence of varicose veins. Researchers naturally conclude that smoking may increase the risk among people predisposed to varicose veins.

**Reconsider the Pill.** Birth control pills raise estrogen levels, as pregnancy does, and may contribute to varicose veins.

**Dress in comfortable clothes.** Avoid tight-fitting clothing, especially snug pants and garters. Any tight garment will create resistance within the circulation and decrease blood flow. It may even cause the blood to be trapped between valves, which could contribute to ballooning of vessels.

**Give your legs a lift.** Dentists, salespeople, barbers and hairdressers all run a higher risk of getting varicose veins, says Dr. De Groot, because they stand on their feet for long hours. The same problem exists for people who sit for long hours; neither group is actually getting any helpful leg exercise. Dr. De Groot recommends that these people take frequent breaks to exercise their legs. "Also, upon getting home from work, such persons should lie on their backs and raise each leg above the level of the heart for a little while. This drains the blood from veins and helps circulation," he says.

**Sit like the boss.** Whenever possible, sit with your feet and legs raised to hip level. Do not sit with your legs crossed at the knee for long periods, nor with your legs folded beneath you. Both postures tend to interfere with circulation.

**Exercise those pumping muscles.** Do some aerobic exercise at least three or four times per week. Walking, swimming or cycling will increase blood circulation by working and strengthening the muscles in your legs. These muscles will pump blood upward and help avoid the development of stagnating pools in the blood vessels.

**Take sun in small doses.** Dr. Goulet warns against getting too much sun. "The sun dilates blood vessels," he says. "Eventually, this can cause them to lose their elasticity. The small capillaries can break, and you have spider veins or worse." Repeated sunburn is particularly dangerous, says Dr. Goulet, because it causes more capillaries to rupture. He also cautions against very hot baths or showers. "Any extreme heat is going to expand blood vessels. Over time, this can hurt them," he says.

## WHEN MEDICAL TREATMENT IS NEEDED

Ask your doctor about the many new procedures for treating varicose veins, including laser therapy, sclerotherapy and new forms of limited surgical techniques. Laser therapy is used to eliminate the smallest capillaries, which usually appear on the face or ankles. Sclerotherapy involves the injection of a chemical substance that irritates the lining of the vein, causing it to collapse and dissolve within the body. Finally, new surgical techniques have been developed that combine ultrasound to limit how much of the vein is removed. "It used to be that the whole vein was removed," says Dr. Goulet, "but now, using new techniques, we are able to be much more precise in how much of the vessel is actually taken out."

Surgeons maintain that there are few, if any, side effects to such procedures. Still, it's best to get at least two opinions about the proper way to deal with your specific concerns.

# 37

# VISION

Sharper, Clearer Eyesight

**Vision** is perhaps the most precious of our senses: It lets us drink in the beauty of a flower, watch the sun set, explore new worlds in novels and movies and look at the people we love.

When vision begins to fade—when the printed word becomes blurry or peripheral vision disappears—it can be pretty upsetting. And as we grow older, the chances of getting a sight-threatening eye disease increase: The three most common eye diseases—glaucoma, cataracts and macular degeneration—affect one of every three Americans older than 65.

But many eye problems are easily remedied, while early treatment can stop some from progressing. And research suggests that some serious eye diseases may be avoided through proper nutrition. Here's the lowdown on eye problems.

## How We See Things

Most eye problems fall under the category of "refractive errors," meaning light rays aren't properly focused on the optic nerve, which sits at the very back of the eye.

Light enters the eye through the cornea—a clear, rounded window—and then passes through a liquid chamber, through the pupil and finally into the lens itself. The cornea, pupil and lens normally contract and expand to focus the light image clearly against the retina. If light is not clearly focused on the optic nerve, the image received by your brain will be blurred or fuzzy.

**A fix for focusing problems.** Myopia, or nearsightedness, is the most common visual refractory error and is caused by a longer-shaped eyeball. Farsightedness, or hyperopia, occurs when the eyeball is shorter than normal. The result is that people have difficulty focusing on close-up objects. For most people, farsightedness gradually decreases with age and often disappears. Both of these conditions can be corrected with glasses or contact lenses. (If you're self-conscious about wearing obvious bifocals, ask your optometrist about "lineless" eyewear.)

Problems focusing close up after the age of 40 is called presbyopia. The lens of the eye loses flexibility as we age and can't focus as well on nearby objects. In most cases, presbyopia can be corrected with simple reading glasses. Those who already have refractive errors—such as myopia or farsightedness—may need bifocals or trifocals to correct for multiple problems.

**Straightening wavy vision.** Astigmatism, another common eye problem, occurs when the cornea has an uneven or rippled surface. Normally, the cornea is smooth and evenly rounded so light is distributed without distortion to the optic nerve. When there are curves on the cornea, the visual image appears wavy. Astigmatism can often be corrected with simple prescription glasses or lenses that correct for the ripples. In some cases, surgery is required.

## TACTICS AGAINST CATARACTS

Cataracts are the gradual clouding and hardening of the eye's lens, making it no longer transparent to light. Vision becomes increasingly hazy and blurred; halos may appear around lights, or you may experience difficulty seeing at night or in bright light. Often, the problems begin in one eye and then progress to the other. Prescription lenses can sometimes compensate. In some cases, surgery may be necessary to remove the defective lens and replace it with a plastic implant that focuses on a set distance.

**Keep 'em covered.** Ultraviolet rays from the sun may contribute to cataracts, so your best bet is to protect your eyes. Wear sunglasses whenever you're outside in the sun; wraparound lenses provide extra protection, and a hat with a brim can help, too. The designation Z80.3 on the sunglasses means they filter out about 95 percent of ultraviolet rays.

**Chow down on beta-carotene.** Beta-carotene, the vegetable source of vitamin A, may prevent the onset of cataracts or slow their formation, says Allen Taylor, Ph.D., director of the laboratory for nutrition and cataract research at the U.S. Department of Agriculture's Human Research Center on Aging at Tufts University in Boston. Beta-carotene, an antioxidant, effectively neutralizes harmful free oxygen molecules that occur in the body and are linked to many degenerative changes.

Studies have shown that people with high blood levels of beta-carotene have significantly lower rates of cataracts, while those people who avoid such foods have higher rates of disease. Good sources of beta-carotene include orange and yellow fruits and vegetables, such as carrots, winter squash, pumpkin, cantaloupe and apricots, as well as dark-green leafy vegetables such as collard greens, kale, and broccoli.

**See what C can do.** In the normal eye, there's a high concentration of vitamin C, according to researchers at Tufts University, while people with cataracts have low concentrations of the vitamin.

In laboratory experiments, vitamin C has been shown to protect the lens from free radical formation, especially that caused by ultraviolet light. Research has shown a strong correlation between high levels of vitamin C and less incidence of cataracts. Dr. Taylor suggests that daily intakes of about 500 milligrams of vitamin C would provide protection against cataracts. That would equal three glasses of orange juice, an ear of corn and a baked sweet potato, for example.

### MOBILIZE AGAINST MACULAR DEGENERATION

The macula is a small area on the center of the retina where cells that detect light and color are tightly packed. These cells begin to break down at about age 60, and straight lines or details begin to appear wavy or distorted. The condition, known as macular degeneration, is the leading cause of blindness in people 75 and over. Laser surgery may be helpful for a few patients.

**Check out your vitamin intake.** In one study, researchers gave daily multivitamins to 192 people with macular degeneration, while another 62 received none. After six months, 33 percent of the supplement group scored better on a vision test, versus 20 percent of the nonsupplement group. Only 22 percent of those receiving supplements got worse, as opposed to 40 percent who didn't get the supplements.

If you want to up your vitamin and mineral intake, your best bet is to eat a balanced diet with a variety of foods, including plenty of fruits and vegetables. If you do choose a supplement, take a balanced multi-vitamin-and-mineral one—overdosing on some nutrients can be dangerous.

**Use the right shades.** Ultraviolet rays may burn and injure the retina and eventually lead to macular degeneration, says Leo Semes, O.D., a consultant to the American Optometric Association and a researcher at the University of Alabama at Birmingham School of Optometry. To prevent or slow down the disease, choose sunglasses with medium- or dark-gray lenses that block ultraviolet rays.

### BATTLE GLAUCOMA WITH REGULAR CHECKUPS

In glaucoma, the pressure inside the eye increases little by little, damaging the blood vessels that feed the retina and optic nerve. The only early warning sign *you* can detect is the gradual loss of peripheral vision.

The illness can be detected during a routine eye exam, however, by measuring the pressure. Medicated eye drops can control and even reduce the pressure inside the eye; sometimes laser surgery is necessary.

Early treatment can halt or slow glaucoma, so it pays to have regular checkups. People in high-risk categories in particular should have annual eye exams, especially after the age of 35. You're at increased risk for glaucoma if you have diabetes, are black, have a parent who had glaucoma or are nearsighted.

MORE TIPS FOR TROUBLED EYES

To keep your eyes comfortable, incorporate these ideas into your daily life.

**Fight dry eyes.** Dry eyes, commonly caused by too much wind, sun or overwork, may also be a side effect of drugs such as diuretics and antidepressants. Blinking, relaxing the eyes or shielding them from wind or light will resolve most dryness— and you should avoid smoke-filled rooms as well as places that are hot and poorly ventilated. You can also use artificial tear drops, available at pharmacies.

**Try a magnifier.** Many people with vision loss can see much better with the use of devices such as magnifying glasses or handheld and stand magnifiers, says Amalia Miranda, O.D., clinical instructor of ophthalmology at the University of Oklahoma Health Sciences Center in Oklahoma City. Other devices available include closed-circuit television that enlarges print on a TV screen and a field enhancer, a prism that increases peripheral vision.

**Think big.** If you have trouble reading, look for large-print books, newspapers and magazines (ask at your local library). You can also buy large playing cards, telephones and clocks with large numbers and high-contrast faces.

## ANTI-AGING CHECKUP
# AN AT-HOME EYE EXAM

When it comes to your eyes, you don't want to ignore any signs of trouble—it could be a problem that could be easily corrected. Answer the following questions Yes or No. Do you:

____ Have particular trouble adjusting to dark rooms, such as at movie theaters?
____ Have difficulty focusing on near or distant objects?
____ Frequently get a new prescription for your glasses or contact lenses—none of which is satisfactory?
____ Squint or blink excessively because of light or glare?
____ Have a change in the color of your iris?
____ Have persistently inflamed or red eyes?
____ Have sudden hazy or blurred vision?
____ Have recurrent pain in or around your eyes?
____ Have double vision?
____ See flashes of light or showers of black spots?
____ See halos or rainbows around light?
____ Have a dark spot at the center of your viewing?
____ See vertical lines as distorted or wavy?
____ Have excess tearing or watery eyes?
____ Have dry eyes with itching or burning?
____ See spots or ghostlike images?
____ Have to turn your head to see things that are beside you? (For example, have you lost peripheral or side vision?)

### INTERPRETING YOUR ANSWERS

If you answered Yes to any of these questions, you should make an appointment for an eye exam. Even if you answered No to every question, however, you should have regular exams, particularly if you have diabetes or a family history of eye problems such as glaucoma or cataracts.

SOURCE: Adapted from "How's Your Vision?: Family Home Eye Test" by the National Society to Prevent Blindness. Copyright © 1988, 1991 by the National Society to Prevent Blindness. Reprinted by permission.

# PART II
## Looking Great

# 38

# AGE SPOTS

### Avoid Those Unwelcome Blotches

**Age** spots—those insidious little "birthday freckles" that seem to pop up overnight—aren't actually related to age at all. They're the result of years of accumulated sun damage.

Age spots are harmless, but they can make us look—or feel—older. Which sort of adds up: The older you are, the more time and opportunity you've had to spend in the sun. So, voilà, you have more "age" spots.

Like freckles and melasma (dark patches that can appear during pregnancy), age spots are caused by too much melanin, the hormone that creates pigmentation beneath the surface of your skin. When repeatedly exposed to the sun, unprotected skin produces too much melanin.

## Spot-Removal Strategies to Try

Not surprisingly, age spots (sometimes called liver spots) generally occur on the face, backs of hands and forearms, where we've gotten the most sun over the years. Chances are, your backside has few, if any, age spots. Here's how to avoid these spots—properly known as solar lentigos—and some options for vanquishing them.

**Double up on sunscreen.** "The only way to stop blotches in their tracks is by sensible sun protection," says Nicholas Lowe, M.D., clinical professor of dermatology at the University of California, Los Angeles, School of Medicine. Experts recommend that you start out with a sunscreen with a sun protection factor (SPF) of 15 or higher to block the sun's ultraviolet rays.

"Apply it to the backs of your hands and to your face first thing in the morning, before you put on any moisturizer or makeup," suggests John E. Wolf, Jr., M.D., professor and chairman of the dermatology department at Baylor College of Medicine in Waco, Texas. "When you wash your hands, don't forget to reapply your sunscreen. If you see the beginnings of age spots or melasma, switch to a higher-SPF sunscreen."

Even people who are conscientious about using sunscreen often apply it too frugally. It takes an ounce or so to cover yourself adequately. Buy two tubes at a time, so you don't run out or skimp.

**Have dubious spots checked out.** If a brown spot does occur suddenly or an old one changes shape, becomes raised or bleeds, have a dermatologist look at it to be certain it's not an early melanoma, or potentially fatal form of skin cancer.

**Shampoo away brown patches.** White- or brown-pigmented areas on your chest, neck or abdomen may not be sun spots at all; rather, they may be caused by a skin condition called *tinea versicolor*. (You'll notice them more in the summer because they don't tan.) Washing the area with a dandruff shampoo that contains selenium sulfide will kill the fungus that causes the problem, and the pigmented areas will disappear. Your physician can prescribe a stronger compound if needed.

**Try an OTC bleaching cream.** If you want to get rid of simple sun spots, the first step is over-the-counter skin-bleaching creams that contain hydroquinone, says Dr. Wolf. Hydroquinone interferes with your skin's production of melanin, so spots don't re-form as your skin sloughs off old layers. These products can take several months or even years to show any improvement, however. (Be sure to wear a sunscreen on top of the bleaching cream.)

"If you try one of the OTC bleaches," says Dr. Wolf, "I recommend you give it a chance for at least a few months. If you see absolutely no difference after using both a bleach and a sunscreen regularly, then you need to go to something stronger." Your dermatologist can prescribe a higher concentration of hydroquinone. This approach works better on light spots than darker areas. You should also be aware that bleaching agents, including hydroquinones, can cause undesirable white, opaque or dark spots on the skin.

---

## ANTI-AGING CHECKUP
## SPOTS THAT WARRANT MORE THAN A GLANCE

Age spots are harmless, but you want to make sure you don't confuse a possibly cancerous skin problem with a sun spot, says Joseph G. Morelli, M.D., assistant professor of dermatology and pediatrics at the University of Colorado Health Sciences Center in Denver. For a suspected age spot—or any spot or growth, for that matter—use the ABCD test, answering each question Yes or No.

_____ A. Shape: Is the spot asymmetrical?
_____ B. Borders: Are the borders irregularly shaped?
_____ C. Color: Is the spot multicolored?
_____ D. Diameter: Is the spot larger than the end of a pencil eraser?

### INTERPRETING YOUR ANSWERS

A. Skin tumors, or melanoma, are often asymmetrical. They're also often raised with an irregular surface. Age spots are flat, and the surface of the skin is normal, except for the discoloration.

B. The border or perimeter of a skin tumor is irregular, raised and clearly defined, as opposed to the flat, often poorly defined border of an age spot.

C. Melanomas are usually multicolored. Age spots are light to darker brown.

D. Melanomas are usually 7 to 10 millimeters in diameter, or about one-fourth to one-third of an inch. Age spots vary in size; some are larger than this, and some are smaller.

If you had any Yes answers, schedule an immediate appointment with a dermatologist to have your spot checked out. Melanomas are a fast-moving form of skin cancer that can be fatal, so don't delay.

**Call in the big guns.** Another option is the use of tretinoin, a vitamin A derivative often used either alone or in combination with hydroquinone to treat acne. Tretinoin—also known as retinoic acid and Retin-A—significantly lightens age spots by inhibiting the production of melanin. A study published in the *New England Journal of Medicine* reported that 20 out of 24 patients using tretinoin experienced significant lightening of age spots after ten months of treatment. The spots didn't return for at least six months after therapy was ended. The people using tretinoin experienced rash and scaliness, however. Some dermatologists have reservations about using this treatment long term, so discuss the pros and cons with your doctor.

**Consider the chemical solution.** Individual spots can be treated with trichloracetic acid, frequently used in chemical peels. "This might be the treatment of choice for someone who has just two or three little spots that aren't too dark," says Dr. Wolf. Another option is freezing the spots with liquid nitrogen. With both of these methods, however, it can be difficult to control the amount of color change that occurs, and the spots can be left too white.

**Have them zapped.** Lasers can destroy the pigmented cells, and the procedure is usually accomplished in one or two visits, depending on the number of spots treated and the darkness of the pigmentation. To treat one age spot the size of the end of a pencil eraser usually takes a few seconds, and the color goes away over the next two to four weeks.

"The great thing about laser treatment for this problem is that in the hands of an expert, you don't run the risk of having white spots where the dark spots had been," says Dr. Lowe. "The only caveat is that, as with any surgery, it's only as good as the practitioner." (Check to make sure the physician is trained in lasers and belongs to the American Society for Laser Medicine and Surgery.)

# 39

# BALDNESS

## A Shrinking Hairline? Don't Panic

**Some** people see baldness as a sign of aging and even a loss of virility, so it isn't surprising that many men view the sight of a receding hairline with a great deal of alarm.

If your hair is disappearing, you're not alone: Millions of American men and women have noticeable hair loss. The most common type, called androgenetic alopecia, can begin as young as age 19 and *is* hormone-linked. Baldness may be associated with higher-than-normal testosterone levels, or hair follicles may simply be genetically predisposed to be more sensitive to hormones that eventually cause the follicles to stop producing hair.

In men, this is known as male pattern baldness. Hair loss begins at the front and back of the head and progresses until the hair on top is completely gone, leaving a horseshoe-shaped ring of hair along the sides of the head. Women may also have this condition, but the thinning occurs much more slowly, and they seldom actually show bald spots.

### POSSIBLE SOLUTIONS

What can you do about disappearing locks?

**First, determine the cause.** Have a checkup to make sure that you don't have an illness or disease that causes hair loss. Although about nine out of ten bald heads are caused by heredity, many factors can cause hair loss, says William A. Bornstein, M.D., Ph.D., clinical assistant professor of endocrinology at Emory University School of Medicine in Atlanta.

Possible causes include crash diets, poor nutrition, pregnancy, oral contraceptives and chronic illnesses such as diabetes and thyroid dysfunction. Shock from illness or a serious operation can result in hair loss up to six or eight months later, and anti-cancer drugs or radiation therapy and even poisoning can result in a loss of hair, either sudden or gradual. In women, high levels of male hormone can cause or contribute to skin problems, excessive body hair and thinning head hair, but this can be treated with drugs, such as spironolactone.

**Preserve your locks with TLC.** Combing or brushing too hard can contribute to hair loss, so take it easy, says John Romano, M.D., a dermatologist at New York Hospital–Cornell Medical Center. First, blot your hair with a towel to remove excess water. Then blow-dry on a low to medium setting, keeping the dryer 6 to 10 inches away from your hair. Use your fingers to place your hair where you want it, then gently style with a wide-toothed comb.

**Make the most of what you've got.** Keep your hair clipped: "The shorter the hair, the denser it looks," advises Gillian Shaw, a barber at Vidal Sassoon in New York. Part your hair slightly off-center. Choose shampoos that make your hair look fuller: Look for terms such as *body-building, thickening* or *volumizing* on the label.

**What about Rogaine?** The drug minoxidil, which is sold under the name of Rogaine, was originally developed to treat high blood pressure. But doctors discovered that for some people, it retards hair loss and even restores hair growth when applied topically.

It's not a wonder drug, however. Eight percent of men using minoxidil experienced moderate or better hair regrowth after 4 months of treatment, says Patrick Guiteras, M.D., clinical faculty member at the University of North Carolina at Chapel Hill School of Medicine, who assessed independent studies on minoxidil. Thirty-nine percent experienced moderate or better regrowth after 12 months. The drug worked best for younger men and for bald spots less than 10 centimeters in diameter that had been hairless for less than ten years.

Minoxidil can work for women as well. Robert L. Rietschel,

M.D., chairman of the department of dermatology at Ochsner Clinic in New Orleans, says he has seen appreciable hair growth in 63 percent of women using minoxidil, even among those age 60.

The key to success is sticking with the program, say proponents. Minoxidil must be applied twice a day for a minimum of four months before you can determine if it's working, states Dr. Guiteras. And it's not cheap: It costs between $40 and $50 a month. If you stop treatments, your regrown hair falls out within a few months.

So far, studies have shown no side effects. People with a history of high blood pressure or heart disease should tell their doctor about these conditions before considering minoxidil, however.

**Tretinoin may give a boost.** "For people who have tried Rogaine and not been impressed with the results but want to keep trying, I might try Rogaine with tretinoin, the acne medication that is also used to treat wrinkles," says Allan L. Kayne, M.D., clinical assistant professor of medicine at the University of Washington and staff dermatologist at the Virginia Mason Clinic, both in Seattle. "In this case, the additional drug may help the Rogaine be absorbed better."

**Get the lowdown on transplants.** A common method of transplanting hair is a punch graft, which moves tiny round plugs of skin with active hair follicles to hairless sites. But advances in technique now allow hairs to be transplanted one or two at a time. "You don't put all the transplanted hairs in a straight line but stagger them, so the results look more natural," says Dr. Kayne.

Using minoxidil may improve the survival rate of the transplanted hairs, says Henry Roenigk, M.D., chairman of the dermatology department at Northwestern University Medical School in Chicago. His studies showed that applying minoxidil for several weeks before and after hair transplants resulted in only a 20 percent loss of transplanted hairs, compared with 50 percent loss when minoxidil wasn't used.

"Cosmetically, hair transplants are one of the most gratifying procedures," says Douglas Altchek, M.D., assistant clinical professor of dermatology at Mount Sinai School of Medicine in New York. "One of my patients, a 39-year-old social worker, had 200 plugs in four months because her thinning hair was embarrassing her. Now, three years later, her hair is growing extremely well, and she's very happy."

## ON THE HORIZON

Currently, minoxidil is the only treatment on the market that can grow new hair or halt hair loss. But in five to ten years, there will likely be more options available, says Douglas Altchek, M.D., assistant clinical professor of dermatology at Mount Sinai School of Medicine in New York. Some treatments being studied:

*Tricomin.* Early results from a study at the University of Rheims in France show that men given high doses of this drug have significant regrowth of hair. In some cases, results were seen in as little as one month.

*Aromatase.* Researchers at the University of Miami isolated this enzyme, which balding men are deficient in. When there's enough aromatase, follicles grow hair; when there's not enough, follicles switch off.

*Electrical stimulation.* Applying low-powered pulses of electrical stimulation to the scalp resulted in new hair or prevented hair loss in 29 out of 30 men in Canadian tests. Their heads were bathed in an electrical current for 12 minutes, twice a week.

*Cyoctol.* One study found that this hormone-blocking drug stopped hair loss or grew hair in 92 percent of the men who used it as a lotion for a year.

*Diazoxide.* Early experiments show that this drug, developed to treat a pancreatic disorder, can also grow hair when applied directly to the head.

(Flap surgery, another kind of hair-transplant procedure, is faster but requires removing wide strips of hair-bearing skin to cover balding areas. In scalp reduction, some of the skin from the scalp is removed and the hair-bearing skin stretched to cover part of the bald area.)

**Or just revise your attitude.** So you're a man and you're going bald. One option is to relax and enjoy it! That's what actor Ted Danson eventually did, revealing his hairpiece on one of the final episodes of *Cheers*.

Losing your hair may not be as bad as you think. In a study reported in the *Journal of Social Psychology*, psychologists asked 29 women and 19 men at the University of Richmond in Virginia for their impressions of composite pictures of men with varying amounts of hair on their heads, with and without beards. The undergraduates were asked to rate each face according to how attractive, intelligent and sociable the man in the picture seemed to be. The students felt that the clean-shaven balding men appeared older but more intelligent, and their opinion of attractiveness wasn't influenced by whether or not they were bald.

If you still have doubts, just look at Sean Connery, selected by *People* magazine as the sexiest man alive, and Patrick Stewart (Jean-Luc Picard of *Star Trek: The Next Generation*), named the most appealing man on television by *TV Guide*. Bald can definitely be beautiful!

**ANTI-AGING CHECKUP**
# ARE YOU BALDNESS-BOUND?

Sometimes it's tough to tell if you're going bald, since hair loss can occur so gradually. To determine if you're heading for baldness, answer these questions Yes or No.

_____ Does your part appear wide or wider than it used to?

_____ Is the number of hairs in your comb or brush increasing, or are there more than 100 a day?

_____ Can you see more scalp than hair when you glance in the mirror?

_____ If you grab a clump of hair and pull firmly, do more than six hairs come out?

_____ If you're a man, are your brothers, uncles or a grandfather bald?

## INTERPRETING YOUR ANSWERS

If you answered Yes to any of these questions, you may want to consider some of the hair-conservation strategies outlined in this chapter.

# 40

# BRITTLE NAILS

Protection for Delicate Nails

**Like** smooth, blotch-free hands, well-kept, healthy fingernails can spell elegance, youth and vitality. But when nails break or chip, they can ruin that elegant appearance.

Why are some nails fragile? "Some people are just born with weak, brittle nails," says Paul Kechijian, M.D., associate professor of dermatology and chief of the nail section at New York University Medical Center. "Then there's another group whose nails become thinner as they get older. There are also the people whose jobs or hobbies cause nail problems." Brittle nails are more common in women and more likely to occur with age.

## BEAUTIFUL NAILS CAN BE YOURS

The good news is that unless your nail problems are caused by a disease such as psoriasis or a thyroid disorder—which require medical care—you can do quite a bit to protect your nails. Here are some of the best ideas professionals have to offer.

**Rehydrate your nails.** Like dry skin, brittle nails suffer from lack of moisture, says Richard K. Scher, M.D., head of the nail section in the department of dermatology at Columbia Presbyterian Medical Center in New York. Cold, dry environments or exposure to harsh chemicals (including some nail-polish removers) can reduce the moisture in nails. To replenish your nails' moisture, soak them at bedtime in luke-warm water for about 15 minutes.

**Slather on moisturizer.** After soaking comes the moisturizer. "If you apply a lotion to your hands as soon as you've lightly dried them, while they're still a bit damp, it helps seal the moisture in your skin and nails," explains Dr. Kechijan. "A moisturizer prevents that rapid expansion and contraction that can cause nails to crack or peel."

"I always tell my clients to apply moisturizer to their hands at least twice a day, before going out in the morning and again at bedtime," says Lia Schorr, of the Lia Schorr Skin Care Salon in New York. For best results, choose a moisturizer with any of the alpha-hydroxy acids, such as lactic acid, glycolic acid and urea.

**Boost nail strength with biotin.** The B vitamin biotin may improve the strength and thickness of nails, according to a Swiss study reported in the *Journal of the American Academy of Dermatology*. Veterinarians often feed biotin to horses to strengthen their hooves, and researchers decided to try it on people with brittle fingernails. In a controlled study of 32 men and women, the researchers gave one group with thin, frail and split nails 2.5 milligrams of biotin daily for six to nine months. Their nails ended up 25 percent thicker.

"Biotin is absorbed into the matrix (supporting structure) of the nail, where it may encourage a better, thicker nail to grow," says Dr. Scher, who treats his brittle-nail patients with biotin supplements.

It's best to check with your doctor before taking supplements, however. There is no recommended daily amount for biotin, but the amount given in the study is considered safe. (Food sources of biotin include cauliflower, soybean flour, lentils, milk and peanut butter.)

**Try some exercise.** Stronger fingers may have stronger nails. "Certain people, such as computer programmers or pianists, subject their nails to chronic, low-grade trauma when they hit the keys," says Dr. Kechijan. "This has been shown to actually stimulate nails to grow a little faster and stronger than they would otherwise." If you don't spend much time at keyboards, you could try drumming your fingers on a table a few minutes every day.

**Use tools, *not* fingernails.** "People should respect their nails more," says Dr. Scher. Nails were never meant to scrape, pry or remove staples, he points out. Also, avoid strong soaps, detergents and excessive hand washing, which alternately stretch and shrink the nail, much like taking a piece of metal and bending it back and forth—eventually it breaks.

**Give yourself an after-bath manicure.** To lessen the possibility of damaging your nails, cut or trim them only after bathing, when they're less brittle.

**Trim and file properly.** Shape your nails with the fine side of an emery board, holding it at a slight angle and filing toward the center. Carry an emery board, and at the first sign of a crack, smooth it away. "You can be doing everything right and still get a little chip in your nail," says Dr. Kechijian. "If you deal with it at once, you can prevent further damage."

**Polish carefully.** Nail polish forms a protective layer and slows down evaporation, says Dr. Scher. Clear polish is best because it shows wear less and hence requires removing less often. (All polish removers can be tough on nails, although those with acetate rather than acetone are less drying.) Try not to change polish more than twice a month; instead, touch it up. When you do apply polish, brush it over the top of your nail, behind the tip, to provide a protective cushion. Wait until your nails are completely dry to apply hand cream or lotion.

**Don't neglect your cuticles.** The rim of skin that borders each nail protects the tissues beneath. If a cuticle is cut or separated from the fingernail, it can expose that area below to bacteria, fungi, viruses and chemicals.

To keep cuticles neat and pliable, soak them in warm water. Do not use a cuticle remover or push back on them, both of which impair the cuticle's ability to protect the finger. Instead, gently massage your cuticles every time you apply your hand cream—they'll be more pliable and less likely to crack.

# 41

# DRY HAIR

## Revitalize Your Parched Tresses

**Imagine,** for a moment, that you're one of those 100,000 or so hairs on the top of your head. First, you spend each night crushed, bent and twisted against the pillow. Morning arrives and before you know it, you're looking up at the nozzle of a shower that's about to pound you with the equivalent of a tropical rain storm. You're wet, cold and flattened, when suddenly you're being blown by a mechanically induced desert wind that feels hot enough to evaporate a small lake. Now you're dry and limp and out the front door, only to be torched by the summer sun or frozen by winter winds. And throughout the day, every time your owner gets nervous, you're the first thing that gets yanked, pulled and twirled.

### OPTIONS TO TRY

Hair can be a beautiful asset, but all too often we abuse it—and the result is dry, brittle, unattractive locks. Here's how you can restore youth, vitality and beauty to your hair.

**If you need to shampoo daily, go ahead.** "Most people who get dry, dull hair think they need to back off from daily washing," says hair expert Philip Kingsley, author of *The Complete Hair Book*. "They're wrong. You can never heal broken hair or split ends, but daily washing and conditioning with good products help to moisturize and elasticize hair."

**Pick the right conditioner.** Conditioners, which help protect hair from outside assaults and repair damage, vary considerably in content. "If your hair is already damaged, it's especially important to choose a conditioner that will counteract your specific problem," says John Corbett, Ph.D., vice president for scientific and technical affairs at Clairol in Stamford, Connecticut. For dry hair, you want conditioners with small amounts of oil: Look for the words *remoisturizer* or *re-elasticizer* on the label or *dimethicone* or *mineral oil* on the list of ingredients. Also, conditioners with low pH factors are better for dry hair.

**Cure flyaway hair.** Static electricity keeps hair from lying smoothly and allows it to tangle more readily. A conditioner will solve this problem. "Your hair naturally has a lot of negative ionic charges along the shaft," says Rebecca Caserio, M.D., clinical assistant professor of dermatology at the University of Pittsburgh. "This causes static. Conditioners add a positive charge, which helps neutralize the static."

**Moisturize through and through.** Twice a week, use a deep-moisturizing conditioning treatment (not an oil treatment) before shampooing, says Kingsley. Ask your beautician to recommend a product that's right for your hair.

**Detangle with care.** Dry hair usually means brittle hair, so you want to take special care when combing. Use a comb with widely spaced teeth on wet hair, and try to untangle snarls with your fingers. Avoid brushing too often.

**Keep the blast to a minimum.** It's best to let your hair dry naturally. If a wash-and-wear style isn't right for you, first blot your hair dry with a towel, then keep your dryer on a low setting at least 6 inches from your head. Keep the dryer moving so the airflow isn't directed at the same spot for more than a few seconds. While your hair is drying, gently finger comb to prevent tangles and stress. (Attaching a diffuser to the nozzle of your blow dryer can also help diffuse hot air more evenly.)

To avoid overdrying sections of your hair, make a part across the back of your head from ear to ear. Comb the upper section of hair forward, and secure it with clips. Start drying at the nape of the neck and work upward toward the crown. When you've dried that section, bring another layer of hair down. Continue working toward the front, and dry the top hairs last.

**Don't sizzle your tresses.** Too-frequent use of curling irons can evaporate the water in the hair shaft that keeps it strong and pliable. This lack of moisture makes hair so brittle, you can damage it by just pulling a comb through it.

---

**ANTI-AGING CHECKUP**
# WHICH SHAMPOO IS RIGHT FOR YOU?

Are you bewildered by the array of different shampoos? Here's a simple guide to choosing the product that's right for you. Your Yes answers will help you narrow down the choices.

____ 1. Do you have coarse hair that isn't excessively oily?

____ 2. Do you have oily hair?

____ 3. Is your hair dry?

____ 4. Has your hair been chemically treated with permanent hair colors, bleaching agents, permanent-wave solutions or straighteners?

## INTERPRETING YOUR ANSWERS

1.  Choose a shampoo for normal hair. Ingredients usually include lauryl sulfate detergents, which offer good cleansing but minimal conditioning. These are fine for adults with coarse hair and moderate oil, but they don't work well for fine or unmanageable hair.
2.  You need a shampoo designed for oily hair, which uses lauryl sulfate and sulfosuccinate detergents. These cleanse well but do not condition. Daily use is not recommended because the detergents can dry the hair shaft.
3.  Dry-hair shampoos reduce static electricity and make fine hair more manageable. Some products provide too much conditioning, which can cause limp hair by letting the conditioner build up on the hair shaft.
4.  Reach for a shampoo for damaged hair, which usually contains mild detergents and stronger conditioners.

If your hair is already damaged, it's best to avoid these tools until your hair has recovered. But styling instruments aren't damaging if they're used properly. And high-quality hair appliances are designed to maintain a certain heat level that helps prevent hair scorching. To avoid damage, don't hold a curling iron in one spot for more than three to five seconds.

**Screen your hair from sun.** The summer months can be especially tough on hair. Protect it from the sun's rays with a scarf, hat or sunscreening conditioner.

**Swimmers need special care.** Swimming in a chlorinated pool can wreak havoc with your hair. The sooner you shampoo after taking a dip, the better. "The chlorine in pools is the same type of chemical used to bleach clothes," says Gary Galante, director of research and development at Chattem Consumer Products. "It forms a bond with the protein in your hair, eventually causing it to break down." To restore overexposed hair, use a shampoo specially formulated to remove chlorine by converting it into water-soluble chloride, which is easily rinsed away.

# 42

# DRY SKIN

Smart Tips for Softer, More Supple Skin

**Soft,** moist skin is more than a matter of comfort. Dewy skin looks healthy, fresh and, yes, *younger.* And moist skin is healthier—the better to protect you against damaging environmental onslaughts.

"It's not just a matter of vanity," says Edward M. Jackson, Ph.D., director of research services and quality assurance at the Andrew Jergens Company. "Dry skin compromises the effectiveness of your skin's barrier against bacteria and other toxins."

Healthy skin is constantly remoisturizing itself, no matter what your age. Water moves up through the top layers of living skin and is redistributed to the uppermost layer of epidermis, which is primarily dead skin. The problem is that this top layer can't hold on to its moisture particularly well. And what little ability it has to hold on to moisture decreases with age.

## MOISTURIZING BASICS

Fortunately, it's possible—and not very complicated—to protect and restore your skin's moisture. Follow these simple tips, and your skin can be youthfully soft and supple year-round.

**Look for water-holding ingredients.** Moisturizers today are better than ever. "Cosmetic science is coming to understand what happens physiologically when a moisturizer interacts with the skin," says Dr. Jackson. "This knowledge is enabling us to duplicate and enhance the materials involved in the process."

The key word is *enhance*. At one time, people believed that water was the key ingredient in a moisturizer, says Charles Fox, cosmetics scientist and independent consultant to the cosmetics industry. "Now we've found that other materials can do the same thing better because they also help hold water." Here are some common ingredients that scientists know are effective.

*Glycerin.* This ingredient seems to stand the test of time. Double-blind clinical trials show that moisturizers containing at least 25 percent glycerin are superior to products without it.

*Lipids.* Lipids are fatty substances that attract, hold and then redistribute the moisture in your skin. Lipids available in moisturizers include cholesterol isostearate and ceramides.

*Petroleum jelly.* Scientists have been taking a second look at this old standby. Once assumed to simply form an impermeable barrier on the surface of the skin, petroleum jelly actually penetrates deeper and helps the skin's natural barrier restore itself.

*Vitamin E.* Some skin-care experts say that vitamin E helps protect the skin because it is an antioxidant—it traps harmful oxygen molecules called free radicals that can damage the skin. "If we can reduce the free radicals, we can delay the aging process a bit," says Fox.

**Treat thirsty skin to AHAs.** "One of the biggest advances in the treatment of dry skin in the last five years has been the use of alpha-hydroxy acids," says Marta Petersen, M.D., assistant professor of medicine at the University of Utah in Salt Lake City. Alpha-hydroxy acids (AHAs) occur naturally in grapes, apples, citrus fruits, sour milk and sugarcane. They not only reduce water loss, prevent thickening of the outer layer of skin and increase the suppleness of the skin, but AHAs also appear to help moisturizers do their job.

One type of AHA, lactic acid, is available over the counter as Lac Hydrin Five and Lacticare. For extremely dry skin, you might try prescription-strength Lac-Hydrin.

## ANTI-AGING CHECKUP
# DO YOU HAVE DRY SKIN?

This quiz not only tells you just how dry your skin really is but also provides you with an instant remedy. Answer the following either Yes or No.

_____ 1. Are your hands in water frequently during the day?
_____ 2. Is your dry, itchy skin aggravated by bathing?
_____ 3. Have you gotten in the habit of mixing bath oil with your bath water?
_____ 4. Do you vigorously scrub your skin when bathing or cleansing?
_____ 5. Is your skin not particularly dry now, but will be come winter?
_____ 6. If it's spring or summer, are you continuing to use the same moisturizer you applied all winter?
_____ 7. Do you live in a city?
_____ 8. Do you consider your skin sensitive?
_____ 9. Do you use a moisturizer every day—but wonder whether it's really working?
_____ 10. Does your skin itch?
_____ 11. Do you have painful, even bleeding, cracks in some areas where your skin is dry?
_____ 12. No matter what products you use, is your skin still dry, red and itchy?

## INTERPRETING YOUR ANSWERS

The more questions you answered Yes, the more of a problem you have with dry skin. But don't despair: Here are the *solutions* to all these problems.

1. Try reducing exposure to water or wearing gloves. Remoisturize often.
2. Take brief, lukewarm baths. Use soap only on the face, armpits, groin and feet; just rinse your torso and extremities with water. Don't scrub!

*continued*

3. If you like the smell of bath oil, that's fine, but it won't do much for your dry skin. It's better to apply a moisturizer immediately after bathing.

4. Scrubbing is a bad idea. Everyone—with or without dry skin—benefits from the gentle technique. Roll the washcloth over your skin; don't rub or scrub.

5. Take preventive action now: Moisturize.

6. As the weather becomes milder, you can switch to a lighter moisturizing lotion.

7. To protect your skin against chemical pollutants in the air, use a moisturizer containing ceramides.

8. When buying a moisturizer, look for the words *nonacnegenic, noncomedogenic, nonallergenic* or *hypo-allergenic* on the label.

9. Skip a day. If your skin still feels supple and not dry, your moisturizer is working.

10. In addition to the tips in this chapter, avoid spicy foods, caffeine and alcohol, all of which can cause dry skin to itch.

11. At bedtime, apply petroleum jelly and cover your hands with thin cotton gloves. The cracks will begin to heal in two to three days.

12. Time to see a dermatologist. You may have an infection or simply need a prescription-strength remedy.

**If it feels good, use it.** Many a dermatologist will tell you that the best moisturizer is the one you like. If it feels good, you'll use it more often, and it will have more opportunity to work. By the way, here's a simple way to tell whether or not your moisturizer is effective: If you miss a day and your skin still feels supple and not dry, it's working.

**Don't wait until your skin feels dry.** Moisturize your skin regularly to *prevent* moisture loss. "This is especially true in winter, when the dry heat inside and the dry cold outside combine to dehydrate even the youngest skin," says Ronald Savin, M.D., clinical professor of dermatology at Yale University.

**Slather on sunscreen.** "The most important thing you can do for your skin is to protect it from the sun," says Nicholas Lowe, M.D., clinical professor of dermatology at the University of California, Los Angeles, School of Medicine. "For this reason, many companies have added sunscreens to their moisturizers."

## SAFEGUARDS AGAINST SUPERDRY SKIN

Regular preventive maintenance can go a long way toward moisturizing dry skin. Here are some additional skin-saver techniques.

**Pull on gloves.** We've all heard about protecting our hands by wearing rubber gloves (preferably latex, with cotton liners) when we have to immerse our hands in water, but how about when you go to bed? "I tell patients to soak their hands in water for five minutes, apply moisturizer, and then put on a pair of clean cotton gloves," says Dr. Petersen. "This helps prevent moisture loss and helps dry skin to heal." You can find these cotton gloves at medical-supply or photo-supply stores.

**Cool it in the tub.** Extra-hot water may feel great, but it's more drying than tepid water, say experts. Although water is a great moisturizer, when it evaporates, it takes your skin's natural moisture with it. And hot water speeds up the evaporation of the skin's essential oils.

**In wintertime, bathe at night.** Showering or bathing before bed gives skin a chance to absorb moisture overnight—which won't happen if you bathe in the morning and then rush right out into the dry, wintry air.

**Pass up the soap.** "Dry skin needs cleansing bars or lotions," says Jeffrey H. Binstock, M.D., assistant clinical professor of dermatologic surgery at the University of California, San Francisco. A waterless liquid cleanser such as Cetaphil or Aquanil applied without water, lathered and then wiped off with a soft cloth may prevent further drying of skin.

**Cleanse only once a day.** If you have oily skin, cleansing twice a day is all right. But if you have dry skin, do it only in the evening. In the morning, just rinse with cool water.

**Apply when wet.** To seal in moisturizer, always apply it to a freshly cleaned face while it's still damp. And don't forget the rest of your body. Using a moisturizer right after bathing or showering seals in your skin's moisture. If you don't use one within half an hour, the water on your skin will evaporate, taking some of your skin's natural oils with it.

**Give trouble spots extra TLC.** Certain areas, such as elbows and feet, may need a heavier moisturizer than hands and face. You may want to wait until bedtime to apply heavier, stickier preparations.

# 43

# FACIAL HAIR

### Say Farewell to Facial Fuzz

**For** most women, it's a well-guarded secret, kept from the most intimate confidants and dealt with behind locked bathroom doors.

No woman wants to admit that she is troubled by facial hair. But it's more common than you probably think: Dark hairs often sprout on the upper lip or chin as women grow older, particularly after menopause. The cause is likely simply heredity or slightly fluctuating hormone levels. Occasionally, excessive hair growth is a sign of some serious underlying disorder involving the ovaries or adrenal glands. If such is the case, other symptoms will send you to your physician.

## WHAT LADIES CAN DO

That said, it's comforting to know that women have various options to cope with facial hair.

**Bleach it.** Bleaching is one of the easiest and most popular approaches. It doesn't remove hair but makes it lighter and less obvious. It's more effective on light growths of light-colored hair. The two most common hair-bleaching agents are hydroquinones and hydrogen peroxide, says Jerald Sklar, M.D., a dermatologist at the Dallas Associated Dermatologists at Baylor University Medical Center. Commercial bleaches designed specifically for facial hair are safer than improvising on your own. It's best to test any preparation on a small area of skin in case you develop a nasty rash. Dab the solution on with a cotton ball, but rinse it away immediately if you feel a burning sensation. Otherwise, apply as directed, and rinse it off after 15 to 30 minutes. Repeat as needed to keep the hair light.

**Prune unwanted growth.** One of the fastest methods to remove unwanted facial hair is clipping it with scissors—or shaving to remove the hair more closely. You can use an electric or regular razor (but you'll want a fresh blade to avoid irritating your face—*not* one you've used on your legs). Shaving won't make the hair darker or thicker, as some people believe, but it will feel stubbly when it grows back. For best results, use a shaving gel and a razor with a pivoting head, says John Romano, M.D., a dermatologist at New York Hospital–Cornell Medical Center.

**Wield the tweezers.** If you have a few errant hairs on your lip or chin, tweezing will do the job. A possible drawback is that the hair may curl under into the skin as it grows back, causing a pimple. If you're plagued by this problem, you'll probably prefer another method of coping with unwanted hair.

Repeated tweezing may eventually destroy the hair follicle, but it may also distort the follicle or cause the hair to grow back thicker. "The tweezing causes blood to rush to the follicle to heal it," resulting in a stronger hair, says Teresa Petricca, president of the American Electrology Association in Trumbull, Connecticut. The only problem is that these conditions can make electrolysis more difficult if you eventually choose that route.

**Wax might work.** The waxing part of this is easy—melted wax is applied to the skin. The *ouch* comes when the wax is hardened and pulled off, taking hair with it. One disadvantage: You have to allow your hair to grow long enough for the wax to get a grip on it.

You won't see new growth again for perhaps several weeks, but waxing, like tweezing, may make the hairs grow in thicker. It can also cause skin irritation and rashes, especially on sensitive skin.

**Consider a chemical.** You can try chemical depilatories specially formulated for the face (those for legs are too harsh). These products remove hair close to the skin and last longer than clipping or shaving. To be safe, it's best to try a depilatory on a small patch of skin, like your inner forearm, before using it on your face, in case you have a reaction to the prod uct. Anything that dissolves hair is pretty potent stuff, so fol low directions carefully. Also, be prepared: These product have a strong odor.

**Zap it away—permanently.** Electrolysis is the only way t permanently get rid of unwanted hair. A needle attached to a electrical source is inserted into the hair follicle, which is the zapped and killed by an electric current. There are two basi techniques: galvanic, the use of electricity to convert body salts to lye, which kills the hair root; and thermolysis, which converts electricity to heat and in turn kills the hair root. Ther are variations on these procedures, and some electrologist combine the two.

Multiple visits are necessary, partly because hair grows i stages. Even if all your existing hairs were successfully elimi nated on the first visit, "resting" follicles in their dorman phase would later produce hair. Also, if hair is particularly thick or has a distorted follicle that is difficult to accurately aim the needle into, it may require several treatments to ki the root.

You'll experience some pain, which varies according to th current used, the area being treated, your own pain threshol and the skill of the electrologist. Costs generally range from $30 to $50 a half-hour. To find the best electrologist in you area, ask your doctor or a local dermatologist for a referral, o write to the American Electrology Association, 106 Oak Ridg Rd., Trumbull, CT 06611.

*Editor's note:* Be sure your operator uses disposable nee dles and sterilized tweezers.

## ANTI-AGING CHECKUP
# IS YOUR HAIR GROWTH NORMAL?

Some facial hair growth in women is normal—particularly in women of Mediterranean descent. Too much, however, could indicate a hormonal imbalance or other health problem, says Jerald Sklar, M.D., a dermatologist at the Dallas Associated Dermatologists at Baylor University Medical Center.

Women have certain amounts of androgens—"male" hormones that include testosterone and androstenedione. Too much can cause masculine hair patterns that include baldness or hair on the face and body. This can be caused by a malfunction or tumor in the adrenal glands or ovaries. Certain drugs, such as prednisone, minoxidil or cyclosporin A, can also spur hair growth.

How much hair growth is too much? Because hair patterns vary from woman to woman, there's no pat answer. But to help you make a determination, check off any of the following conditions that apply to you.

_____ A change in menstrual cycle, including irregular periods

_____ Body and facial hair that becomes thicker and coarser

_____ Body hair that begins to appear in unusual areas such as the stomach or chest

_____ A previous diagnosis of polycystic ovary disease

_____ Unintentional increase in muscle mass, unrelated to resistance training

_____ A deepening voice

### INTERPRETING YOUR ANSWERS

If you have checked off any of these conditions, make an appointment with your physician or an endocrinologist. Some problems can be treated simply with hormones or with spironolactone, a drug that counteracts the side effects of excessive androgen.

# 44

# GRAY HAIR

Color Options That Make Sense

**They** creep up on you: first one, then a few more. Before you know it, your hair is streaked with silver.

What do you do about gray hair? What you *don't* do is despair. Some people look great in silvery tresses, like Heloise, author of the "Hints from Heloise" column, who began to gray when she was very young. Others—about half of all women over 40 (and many men), in fact—decide to color or disguise the gray with a variety of coloring agents.

### WHAT'S YOUR BEST ALTERNATIVE?

Whatever you choose, you want to look your best. Here are some options.

**Love that gray!** You need to treat gray hair with special care: Always use a conditioner, advises Nick Berardi, a senior hairstylist for Vidal Sassoon in New York, because gray hairs tend to be coarser than other hairs. You should also work with your stylist to choose a style that's the most flattering. Although Heloise looks great with her long gray hair, most women with gray hair look best with it cut above the shoulders, says Berardi. Also, gray hair is often wiry and responds better to a shorter style.

**Choose the right coloring process.** If you decide you want to disguise your gray hairs, you have plenty of products to choose from. There are six types: temporary rinses, semipermanent colors, permanent oxidation dyes, lead acetate dyes, vegetable dyes and highlighting. Here's the lowdown on these methods.

*Temporary rinses.* These are somewhat like a coat of paint: The color sits on the hair surface and comes off when you shampoo, so it's a good way to test a color. The dyes are usually synthetic and have been tested for safety by the Food and Drug Administration (FDA).

---

## WHEN GRAY HAIR ISN'T PERMANENT

For most of us, gray hair is a natural and unstoppable result of aging. Eventually, some or all of the hair follicles stop producing pigment; how soon and how much depends on genetics.

But occasionally, gray hair may result from a disease or even a physical or mental shock. Endocrine gland disorders, nervous system disorders, vitiligo and malaria can all cause your hair follicles to stop producing pigment. In these cases, the color change may be temporary, and color may return as new hair grows in.

---

*Semipermanent colors.* A semipermanent formula washes out after four or five shampoos—so you're not stuck with a color you don't like. Both gray and colored hair will be dyed, however, so choose a shade lighter than your original color to avoid unnatural contrasts, suggests John Corbett, Ph.D., vice president for scientific and technical affairs at Clairol in Stamford, Connecticut.

*Permanent oxidation dyes.* You can buy at-home kits for permanent dyes, but as the hair grows out, the new growth needs to be retouched, and this is best done by a professional. (If you re-dye all the hair to cover the new growth, you'll get too much color built up on the "old" hair.) These dyes are the most likely to cause allergic skin reactions.

*Lead acetate dyes.* These products, used mostly by men, are applied progressively—combed in daily until the desired color is achieved. This color is tough to remove, tends to dull the appearance of the hair and produces a dark color.

*Natural dyes.* Commonly called vegetable dyes, these products once included various plants and even extracts from wood. Today dye made from henna is the only natural dye available, and it's limited to various shades of brown and red. It needs to be reapplied every two to three months.

*Highlighting.* This process lightens strands of hairs for a "streaked" effect with various colors that help disguise the gray. It's best for people with dark blond or brown hair and lasts from three to six months.

**Find a good stylist.** You can buy all kinds of hair-coloring products for at-home use, but making drastic color changes or applying permanent dyes is best left to professionals. To find a good stylist, ask for recommendations from friends who have hair similar to yours. Talk to the stylist and, if possible, watch him or her work before committing yourself.

**Before using dyes, test for reactions.** Some people have adverse reactions to hair-coloring products, and dermatologists recommend that you always try this patch test.

1. Thoroughly wash the crease on the inside of your elbow, and dry it.
2. Wet a cotton swab with the hair-coloring formula, and dab it on the patch of skin that you just washed. The dab should be at least as big as a quarter.
3. Wait between 24 and 48 hours to see if the skin shows irritation or an allergic reaction such as redness, rash, irritation, itching or pain.

**Minimize the risks.** Many common coloring products, especially those made of derivatives of coal tar and petroleum, contain chemicals that have been linked to cancer. In addition, the progressive agents contain lead, a highly toxic metal, says John Bailey, Ph.D., acting director of the FDA's Office of Cosmetics and Colors in Washington, D.C.

Research reported in the *American Journal of Public Health* has suggested a link between hair dyes and an increased risk of leukemia, multiple myeloma and non-Hodgkin's lymphoma. Risks were higher among women who used darker shades—brown, black or red—of permanent hair colors.

All hair dyes enter the skin to some extent and can migrate

to the bloodstream, says Dr. Bailey. However, the amounts that ultimately do make their way into the blood are minute and appear to be too small to have an effect. To minimize possible risk, follow the directions carefully and avoid contact with the eyes or any open cut. You may also want to choose lighter, temporary shades, rather than darker, permanent ones. And to lessen the chance of getting the dye in their mouths, men should not use lead-containing dyes on beards or mustaches.

## ANTI-AGING CHECKUP
# IS YOUR HAIR COLOR RIGHT FOR YOU?

If you choose to color your hair, for best results, select a color that's closest to your original, natural shade, says John Corbett, Ph.D., vice president for scientific and technical affairs at Clairol in Stamford, Connecticut. Also, keep in mind the color of your skin when coloring your hair. As men and women pass the age of 40, lighter shades create less contrast between hair and skin; dark shades are too harsh and accentuate less-than-perfect skin.

To select the most flattering hair color, answer these questions Yes or No and refer to the guidelines below.

_____ 1. Do you have olive skin and dark hair?
_____ 2. Do you have light or reddish skin and brown or red hair?
_____ 3. Do you have black or dark brown skin and dark hair?
_____ 4. Are you blond?
_____ 5. Is your hair less than 20 percent gray?

### INTERPRETING YOUR ANSWERS

1. If this describes you, you should probably stick with your original color, or lighten it with a soft medium brown or medium ash. Ash has no red shades, which might conflict with olive skin.
2. People who fit this description can use an auburn color, with light-red highlights, or burgundy, which has subtle purple or violet undertones. People with this combination can also use henna, a natural coloring agent that will wash out.
3. If you have dark hair and dark skin, you can color the gray or lighten your hair to brown or lighter shades of brown.
4. If 40 percent or more of your hair is gray, a permanent color that covers gray without changing the existing colored hair is probably best. Don't use peroxide-containing formulas because they will lighten existing color.
5. Choose a shade lighter than your natural color.

# 45

# LIPS

Tips for Terrific Lips

**You** can pucker up all you want, but the most alluring smile quickly loses it appeal when your lips are cracked, peeling and dry.

Your lips suffer even more than other delicate facial skin from the sun and the weather. Unlike the rest of your skin, lips contain no melanin and lack oil glands to protect against drying winds and indoor heating. Sun damage also speeds up the formation of those pesky vertical lines that lipstick can seep into.

But take heart: Luscious lips can be yours! All you need is a little bit of daily care to keep your mouth its most attractive. Here are some expert tips to help you keep your lips plump, moist and full.

**If you lick your lips, stop.** As natural as it may seem, licking your lips only makes dry lips drier. "This is one of the very worst things people can do," says Ronald Sherman, M.D., senior clinical instructor in dermatology at Mount Sinai Medical Center in New York. "It only increases evaporation. When the moisture from licking your lips evaporates, so does some of the moisture from your lips." Furthermore, saliva contains drying enzymes.

**Slick on a mouth-watering balm.** The *right* way to protect your lips against sun and weather is to moisturize them with lip balms with sunscreen. Apply day and night and reapply often, especially after meals, before going outside and at bedtime. If your lips are naturally dry, dab a drop of water on

267

them before applying lip balm, so the oils in the balm can seal in the moisture.

**Clever tricks for fuller lips.** For women who yearn for the fuller-lipped look that keeps the smile youthful, makeup can work wonders.

**Start with a good base.** Even the healthiest lips will be ruined by cakey or poorly applied lip color. To color yourself gorgeous, apply a lip conditioner, then a foundation base. This will help your lipstick go on evenly.

**Use a lip pencil for definition.** To prevent feathering, the less-than-stylist effect you get when lipstick seeps into the vertical lines that extend beyond your lips, use a neutral-colored lip pencil to neatly outline and fill in your lip line. Pencils not only help prevent lipstick color from bleeding, they also allow you to make minor alterations in your natural lip line. "The number one thing to remember is that a lip pencil should be used to give definition only," says beauty expert Trish McEvoy of New York. "Look for a shade close to your natural lip color. Angle the pencil (or use one with a rounded tip) to shape the lips symmetrically, yet keep the line soft (using the point can create a harsh appearance). For the most flattering look, simply follow your own lip line." She suggests you blend the line with a swab until it's barely noticeable.

**Try pencils of different consistencies.** Pencils that are too soft bleed as badly as lipstick, while those that are too hard pull the lip and give a choppy line. When shopping, try the tester on the back of your hand. "If the temperature of the store you're in is cool, warm the pencil tip a bit by drawing on your hand," McEvoy suggests. "Cold can make even the best formulas stubborn." Then lightly try to rub off the lip pencil. If it disappears from your hand, it won't last on your lips. And if the pencil drags or skips, forget it.

**Choose the right finish.** Next, fill in your outlined lips with color. The best lipsticks for most women are matte creams. They're least likely to irritate, and they last longer than frosts, which call attention to chapping and are less flattering on mature women. Glosses tend to wear off quickly.

**Brush on color.** No matter which type of color you choose, apply it with a lip brush, at least for the first application of the day. "Then you'll only need to touch up by placing color within the outline during the day," says McEvoy. Be sure to apply color evenly, keeping it inside the lip line. Work from the center of your mouth outward. When you're done, give your lips a light dusting of face powder, and blot gently with a tissue to set the color.

---

## ANTI-AGING CHECKUP
# TROUBLESHOOTING LIP PROBLEMS

Here's a checklist of lip problems. Answer Yes or No to each.

_____ 1. Do you spend a lot of time outdoors?

_____ 2. Do you lick your lips?

_____ 3. Are your lips so chapped that they're cracked?

_____ 4. Do you always have trouble getting your lipstick to go on evenly?

_____ 5. Does your lipstick bleed?

_____ 6. Do you dislike your lip line?

_____ 7. Have you ever tried a lip pencil and found that it made a mess?

_____ 8. Does your lipstick fade?

_____ 9. Do you bite your lips?

_____ 10. Do your lip problems refuse to improve or go away?

### INTERPRETING YOUR ANSWERS

If you answered Yes to any of these questions, here are some solutions to your problems.

1. Use a sunscreen to protect your lips from sun damage.
2. This is an indication that your lips are too dry. Moisturize with a lip balm and apply a drop of water first.
3. You need a medicated lip balm with sunscreen.
4. Apply a lip conditioner, then a foundation base. This will help your lipstick go on evenly.
5. Use a lip pencil to define the line.
6. Get out that lip pencil again. Use it to make minor improvements in your lip line.

*continued*

7. The pencil was probably too soft. When you shop for a lip pencil, try it out on the back of your hand first before you buy it.

8. Chances are you're not applying it often enough. It's important to find a lip product with a "feel" you like. That way, you'll have no problem reapplying it often, especially after meals, before going outside and at bedtime.

9. Stop! Biting your lips is even worse than licking them. It removes protective skin.

10. Time for a visit to your dermatologist. Persistent problems may require medical care.

**Don't rub.** Never rub off your lipstick. Rubbing removes protective surface cells. If you need to remove your lipstick for any reason, blot it off.

### ABOUT THOSE WHISTLE LINES . . .

If simple care and makeup don't resolve your lip problems, there are two procedures you can ask your doctor or dermatologist about.

Retin-A, a vitamin A derivative, may help lips look younger. "Retin-A can also help with fine wrinkling around the lips," says Marta Petersen, M.D., assistant professor of medicine at the University of Utah in Salt Lake City. Originally developed as an anti-acne medication, patients who used Retin-A discovered that it brought about an overall improvement in minor wrinkling and age spots.

If your lines are too deep to camouflage, they can be plumped up with the injection of collagen, the fibrous protein in skin that keeps it from drooping and sagging. "Collagen injections can help a great deal," says Dr. Sherman. The procedure is approved by the Food and Drug Administration, he points out, and all that's required is that you have a skin test beforehand to be sure you're not allergic to the collagen.

Note that because the lip area is sensitive, there will be discomfort during the procedure. And the area will be puffy for a few hours afterward—though makeup can help disguise that. The injections need to be repeated every six months or so because the collagen is gradually absorbed by the body.

# 46

# SKIN FLAWS

## How to Look Ten Years Younger

**Is** anything more off-putting than someone asking if you're feeling ill when you're actually feeling great—or you *were?* Well, here's how you can prevent looking tired and older than your age—or even looking your age at all. All of these tips have the goal of restoring health and vitality to your appearance, but looking good isn't a question of vanity. When you know you look great, *feeling* great often follows.

### ERASE CIRCLES AND PUFFINESS

Fatigue often shows first on the delicate skin around the eyes. Puffiness and circles conspire to make us look our oldest, and some people are born with a tendency toward these.

"For many people, it's possible to prevent or greatly reduce puffiness, especially the kind that's worse in the morning as a result of overnight fluid retention," says Fredric Haberman, M.D., clinical instructor of medicine at Albert Einstein College of Medicine in New York and author of *The Doctor's Beauty Hotline*. Here are a few of Dr. Haberman's suggestions.

**Change your position.** Sleep on your back or with your head elevated by several pillows to keep fluid from pooling around your eyes while you sleep. You can even put two or three folded blankets under your mattress, at the head of your bed, to elevate your head.

**Consider allergies.** If you use a down comforter or pillow, try switching to a different type.

**Splash away puffiness.** If you still have residual puffiness, try splashing your face several times with cold water to help stimulate the circulation away from your eyes.

**Try tea bags.** Lia Schorr, of the Lia Schorr Skin Care Salon in New York, suggests this tactic: Soak four tea bags in luke-warm water, then apply two to each eye. If it's circles that are your beauty bête noire, use a concealer patted gently around your eye, from the bone toward the lash line.

## ERASE STRESS

If you look at yourself in the mirror at lunch and there's an older stranger with hunched shoulders and a furrowed brow staring back, don't just tell yourself you need a vacation. Instead, take a few minutes to unwind and get your body back to normal.

**Cool off.** Run a clean cloth (or paper towel) under cool water. Cover your eyes with tissue, and blot your face all over with the cloth.

**Relax.** Sit comfortably with both feet on the floor. Tell your body to relax your shoulders. Tilt your head back slightly, and lower your jaw as far as you can. Then relax your jaw and allow it to raise naturally.

**Bob a bit.** Bend your body toward the floor as far as you can, then gently bob up and down from the waist for a few minutes with your neck, arms and hands totally relaxed.

**Take a stroll.** Get outside for five minutes and breathe some fresh air.

**Practice good posture.** This may seem more like something you tell a teenager: "Don't slouch," or "Pick your feet up when you walk." But an upright stance and an easy, graceful carriage can make everyone look their best and most youthful. One exercise that's particularly good—you can do it anywhere, anytime—is to picture a thread that goes through the center of you and holds you up. If you can imagine it extending through the center of your head and pulling you back into alignment, you can get out of the habit of slumping.

### Pamper Your Face and Hands

Your hands and face are always there for people to notice and judge, so don't let age spots and roughened skin create the wrong impression.

**Give yourself a face-lift.** The quickest and most convenient anti-aging ploy you can use is to smile. A smile not only draws your features upward, it's a facial expression of youth and creates a positive impression.

**Use sunscreen.** Prevent age spots by applying a sunscreen to your face and hands every morning, again at lunch and every time you wash your hands. Today's moisturizers with sunscreen allow you to fight age spots and rough skin at the same time. Be sure that the product you use contains a sunscreen with a sun protection factor (SPF) of at least 15 for adequate protection. (Even if you wear sunscreen, it's a good idea to protect yourself from too much sun because sunscreens can't block *all* rays.)

**Try a mask.** Nothing says old and tired like dull, flaky, lifeless-looking skin. A great temporary remedy for this is a mask. "Masks can provide gentle exfoliation and moisture benefits, too," says Schorr. For dry skin, just whip up the yolk of one large egg and smooth it on your face and throat. (If you want to give your hands a similar treat, you need another egg.) After five to ten minutes, rinse with cotton pads soaked in lukewarm water. "Yogurt is another great facial mask," says Schorr. You can also buy mask preparations in a drugstore or department store.

After you've completely removed the mask, follow with an all-over application of your favorite moisturizer to help your skin stay soft. Don't forget to treat the rest of your skin with a moisturizer if it needs it. Maintaining soft and smooth skin doesn't stop at your jawline.

### Makeup Tips to Erase Years

With the right makeup techniques, you can give your face a younger appearance.

**Apply a good foundation.** Young skin has a smooth, even color. To re-create this, use a tinted moisturizer on your face and throat, or a regular moisturizer followed by a lightweight foundation that matches your skin color. The shade should be only a little darker than your own.

This whole process takes just two minutes, and you can minimize patchy pigment and present a smooth face to the world. To help prevent further dark spots, use a moisturizer that contains an SPF of 15 or higher.

**Use a blusher.** As we mature, our circulation sometimes slows down, which can, in turn, leave us looking a bit washed out. We still associate a touch of color with the healthy vitality of youth.

The two critical considerations when applying blush are replacement and blending. You can usually wear any shade you want, as long as it's applied correctly. We've all seen women with round spots of strong cheek color that make them look like Kewpie dolls. Generally, look for a nonfrosted shade to complement your lipstick and your skin tone.

For a beautiful, natural application, start on the apple of your cheek (smile at yourself in the mirror to locate the apples), and smooth your blusher toward your hairline. When you're finished, the result should be a seamless wash of color on your cheeks. If you see lines, use a cotton pad to gently buff them away.

**Pay attention to your brow line.** Perfect eyebrows would be in proportion to the rest of your features, match your coloring and sweep up and out at the tips to avoid "dragging down" the rest of your face. For most of us, nature fails us in at least one of these regards. So help nature along. "First, use an eyebrow brush or a toothbrush to brush the hairs up, toward your hairline," says Schorr. Next, fill in with a soft neutral, light-brown or blond pencil for the most natural look. Use short, feathery strokes.

A little technique that makes a big difference: To help downward-growing hairs stay swept upward, finish by stroking over them with an old toothbrush, then set with clear mascara.

# 47

# SPIDER VEINS

### Banish These Unwanted Webs

**They're** aptly named, those blue, red or purple webs of tiny capillaries that sometimes show up on the face and legs.

While spider veins might annoy you, they shouldn't alarm you. Spider veins (also called telangiectasias) are not dangerous or a sign of illness but are merely overgrown, dilated blood vessels. Unlike their larger, bulgy cousins, varicose veins, spider veins aren't painful. What's more, they're *not* an inevitable sign of aging—teenagers can get them, too. (They do, however, tend to be more common the older you get.) "Very few women over 30 do not have some spider veins on their legs," says Arthur P. Bertolino, M.D., Ph.D., associate clinical professor of dermatology at the New York University Medical Center.

Men get spider veins, too, but they're more common in women, which suggests a link to hormone levels. And, in fact, puberty, pregnancy, birth control pills, estrogen replacement therapy and other hormonal imbalances can make them worse.

### First, Discourage Those Tiny Veins

Spider veins may not be harmful or painful, but many people consider them, well, *unsightly*. Fortunately, you don't have to live with spider veins. Here are some tips to help avoid them.

**Steer clear of sun and steam.** Spider veins are a major sign of sun damage, says Marta Petersen, M.D., assistant professor of medicine at the University of Utah in Salt Lake City. No one knows whether the sun directly triggers the abnormal growth of the blood vessels or whether the abnormal growth is a result of the skin trying to repair itself, she says.

Wear a wide-brimmed hat out-of-doors, recommends Jonathan K. Wilkin, M.D., director of the division of dermatology at the University Hospital Clinic in Columbus, Ohio. Also, use a sunscreen with a sun protection factor of 15 or above year-round. Because heat can cause blood vessels to dilate, stay out of steam rooms and saunas.

**Protect your face from the wind and cold.** When outdoors in the cold, protect your face with a scarf or mask, suggests Dr. Wilkin. You could also smear a layer of petroleum jelly on your nose to help protect it.

**Try support hose.** Standing for long hours can definitely contribute to spider veins on the legs, and support hose *may* help prevent them, says Dr. Petersen. If your profession requires a lot of standing, you may want to try these hose.

**Wear comfortable clothing.** Doctors suggest that tight clothing and girdles can make spider veins worse by impairing circulation. Loosening up your wardrobe could make a difference, says Dr. Bertolino. That means fuller-cut jeans and no cinch-waist belts, for instance.

**Ask your dermatologist about rosacea.** Spider veins are one symptom of rosacea, a skin problem that most commonly occurs in the 30s and 40s in fair-skinned people prone to blushing. Other symptoms can include flushing and redness, acne-like outbreaks or red, knobby bumps on the nose. A dermatologist can prescribe oral and topical medications to help control the rosacea and prevent it from progressing.

**Make your favorite drink alcohol-free.** Drinking alcohol doesn't *cause* spider veins or rosacea, explains Dr. Wilkin, but it can make them worse. How much is too much? Determine by trial and error: In some people, two glasses of wine are enough to make the face flush and turn the nose reddish.

**Go easy on spicy foods.** If hot chicken wings and spicy chili cause your face to redden, steer clear of them. Avoid *any* spicy food that elicits such a reaction.

**Tepid is better than scalding.** This includes steaming-hot coffee and soup. Doctors once believed that caffeine was the problem but now agree that it is the *heat* from coffee, and not the caffeine. This doesn't mean you have to go without soup or coffee—just let it cool slightly before eating or drinking. Or plop an ice cube in your bowl or cup.

**Reconsider your birth control method.** Hormonal imbalances, which sometimes occur with oral contraceptives, can cause spider veins. If your spider veins appeared after you started the Pill, there might be a connection, according to Brian McDonagh, M.D., a vein specialist in Chicago and founder and director of Vein Clinics of America. Ask your physician: You may want to try a Pill with a different formulation or use a different method of birth control.

### LASERS AND OTHER ANTI-SPIDER-VEIN MARVELS

To remove spider veins requires the services of a dermatologist—preferably a physician skilled in the best techniques. Ask your physician for a referral, or call a few dermatologists and ask how often they treat these pesky little veins. "Dermatologists who do these procedures often are good at it and can do a better job," says Dr. Petersen.

**Eradicate with sclerotherapy.** Sclerotherapy is the treatment of choice for spider veins on the legs. A special solution is injected into the spider veins with a very fine needle. "The solution irritates the vessel's lining, causing it to stick together and eventually collapse," says Dr. Bertolino. "Within two or three weeks, the spider vein becomes scar tissue and eventually disappears."

Dr. Bertolino says people who undergo sclerotherapy can expect about 80 percent improvement. "The procedure is done in the office, and patients can walk out moments later," he says. The number of treatments depends on the number of veins and their size. Side effects, though rare, include bruising, brown spots, swelling and ulceration. "Sclerotherapy is one of the safest procedures in cosmetic dermatology," adds Dr. Bertolino. "And it often has wonderful psychological rewards. People look better, so they feel better about themselves."

If you decide to go this route, ask your doctor about Polidocanol, a European drug used in sclerotherapy. "The dermatologists who use it say it's much better than saline solution," says

Dr. Petersen. "There's much less discomfort—almost none at all—and the risks of side effects are fewer." Dr. Petersen points out that Polidocanol has not yet been approved by the Food and Drug Administration. Check with your dermatologist for updates.

**Zap spider veins on the face.** The smaller veins on the face present a greater challenge. It's more difficult to inject a solution into such a small target, so the likelihood of side effects is greater. A preferred treatment is copper vapor laser therapy. Because of the particular wavelength of the laser, the spider veins absorb it more readily than the surrounding tissue. The tiny blood vessels are destroyed, but nothing else. "It's not painless," says Dr. Petersen, "but it works pretty well on the face and seems to have less of a damaging effect on the top layer of skin."

Another form of electrotherapy, galvanic current therapy—in which an electric current is applied by injection—was once the standard for treating spider veins on the face, according to Dr. Bertolino. Laser therapy is more effective and has less chance of requiring retreatment, however.

# WHAT TO DO FOR CHERRY ANGIOMAS

What? You've never heard of a cherry angioma? Chances are you've met plenty of people who have one or more—and perhaps you do, too. Most people just don't know what they're called.

Cherry angiomas are small, bright-red spots or mounds, often about the size of the head of a pin or a bit larger. They're most common on the stomach, back, arms or chest, although they could appear just about anywhere. Tiny though they may be, cherry angiomas are composed of hundreds of dilated capillaries clumping on the skin surface and are completely harmless. While technically not a sign of aging—they can occur at any time—they do tend to be more common as we grow older.

If these vermilion speckles don't bother you, ignore them, advises Marta Petersen, M.D., assistant professor of medicine at the University of Utah in Salt Lake City. "Most of the time, people with cherry angiomas opt for no treatment at all," she says. "Cosmetically, they're not too disturbing, since they're usually on the trunk."

If they *do* bother you, cherry angiomas can be removed via a procedure called electrodesiccation. An electrical instrument sends a small charge into the treated veins, dehydrating and destroying them. Ask your dermatologist for details.

# 48

# TEETH AND GUMS

A Brilliant Smile—For Keeps

**There** was a time, not too long ago, when gum disease—also called periodontal disease—was generally considered an inevitable part of aging: Get older; lose your teeth. And the unfortunate truth is that inflammation and infection of the gums and bone supporting the teeth is still the most common cause of tooth loss in adults.

The good news is that with proper care, not only can you keep your natural teeth, gums and supporting jawbone for a lifetime, you can preserve—and even enhance—the youthful strength and gleam of your teeth. Periodontal disease can be prevented. And if it should develop, it can be effectively treated. "Dentures will become archaic. The picture of the grandparents with their teeth in a glass in the bathroom will be gone," predicts Geraldine Morrow, D.M.D., member of the American Association of Women Dentists.

Even if you do lose an occasional chopper to disease or injury, you may never need removable dentures. Modern techniques now available to replace lost teeth can keep your smile healthy and bright.

### PRACTICE YOUR PREVENTIVE POWERS

Exactly what are you preventing—cavities? Gum inflammation? Infection?

All three, actually. Strategies for preventing cavities prevent gum disease, too. Here are some at-home tips.

**Give yourself quality toothbrush time.** You can rest assured that you're doing a thorough job of brushing and flossing if you spend at least five full minutes at it every day. Spread your brushing time over two or three sessions; it is more effective that way.

**Get the right angle on brushing.** The root cause of periodontal disease is plaque, a sticky buildup that accumulates at the gum line. To get at the plaque below the gum line, where it's most dangerous, start by holding the brush horizontal to your teeth. Then rotate it so the brush ends point upward toward the gum line for top teeth, downward for bottom teeth, at about a 45-degree angle. Then brush, using circular strokes, working the bristles into the crevices between teeth and gums—with gentle pressure and short strokes.

**Fortify teeth with fluoride.** Topical fluoride helps shore up tooth enamel and strengthens root surfaces, which is especially helpful in preventing root decay and root sensitivity. So use fluoride toothpaste or a rinse containing fluoride. And if your teeth are sensitive, use a fluoride-containing toothpaste made for sensitive teeth.

**Learn to saw through plaque.** Adults and children over age 10 should floss at least once daily, preferably twice. (For younger children, an adult should do the flossing.) A gentle sawing motion works best: When the floss reaches the gum lines, curve it into a C-shape against one tooth. Carefully slide it into the space between the gum and the tooth until you feel resistance. Gently scrape the side of the tooth while moving the floss away from the gum. Be sure to follow these steps on both sides of all your teeth, even the ones way in back. Then rinse with water to remove debris loosened by flossing.

**Use waxed floss for tight places.** Waxed or partially waxed floss is least likely to shred, so it's best for squeezing between crowded or crooked teeth. Extra-thick floss or dental tape cleans large spaces. If you have problems working with your fingers or have hard-to-reach areas, try using a dental-floss holder (available in most drugstores).

**Try some vitamin C for bleeding gums.** Bleeding gums are a red flag for gum disease. The number one remedy is proper brushing and flossing, but low body levels of vitamin C can make the problem worse. "The severity of gum disease and the rate at which it progresses is definitely related to a lack of nutrients, like vitamin C," says Winston Morris, D.M.D., a specialist in endodontics and orthodontics and coauthor of *The Balanced Nutrition Plan for Dental Patients*.

### HIGH-TECH SMILE SAVERS

Despite the most conscientious efforts, "bacteria can sometimes escape even the best home care and gain a foothold under your gums," says Michael G. Newman, D.D.S., a professor at the University of California, Los Angeles, Dental School. And other problems can occur: Your teeth may be stained, chipped or crooked. But dentists, periodontists and other dental professionals are there to save your smile. Here are the various ways they can help.

**Take your teeth to the cleaners.** A thorough cleaning at the dentist's office can remove not only plaque and tartar but a lot of tooth discoloration as well. Professional cleaning invigorates your gums, too.

**Press on porcelain.** Think of porcelain laminates (veneers) as press-on fingernails for your teeth. Though more expensive than a similar procedure called composite bonding, veneers are more durable and probably last longer—10 to 12 years. The front of the tooth is painted with adhesive, then the veneer pressed into place.

**Brace yourself.** There really is no age limit for orthodontic treatment. And while the cosmetic and psychological pluses are often reason enough for braces, health benefits add to their appeal. Since crowded or misaligned teeth are tougher to clean, proper realignment may help prevent gum disease, decay and eventual tooth loss. Braces may also limit or reverse gum disease that's already brewing.

**Look into lifelike crowns.** If a crown is required to repair a damaged or misshapen tooth, ask your dentist about using one of the good-looking new porcelains. "It used to be that the metal substructure always made the crown look artificial," says Barry G. Dale, D.M.D., a cosmetic and general dentist in Englewood, New Jersey. "But the new porcelains provide close to, if not the same, lifelike quality of your natural teeth."

**Flash a Teflon smile.** Well, not really. The Teflon is used as an implant to help rebuild lost bone and ligament. The compound serves to keep gum tissue from collapsing on the gap left by the lost bone. The shield guides the tissue in regenerating new, stronger root surface, ligament and bone. If you have moderate to severe bone loss at some point in your jaw, your doctor may suggest a specialist in this technique, which is called guided tissue regeneration.

**Feel whole again with implants.** Ask your dentist if implants are right for you. By setting a sort of artificial root into your jawbone, the dentist may be able to attach your new tooth to this anchor, which doesn't depend on the surrounding teeth, as do bridges. "Implants—because they're fixed in your mouth so only a dentist can remove them—are akin to having your own teeth," says Albert D. Guckes, D.D.S., deputy clinical director of the National Institute of Dental Research, a branch of the National Institutes of Health.

---

### ANTI-AGING CHECKUP
## OPEN WIDE AND LOOK INSIDE

Your dentist is the best person to evaluate the condition of your teeth and gums. But you can and should be on the lookout for signs that some extra care is needed for your pearly whites and their supporting cast.

First, to check how well you're brushing your teeth, chew on a disclosing tablet, then rinse. These little wonders, available at drugstores, contain a harmless dye that stains plaque red and lets you know where you need to concentrate more effort when brushing.

Answer these three questions Yes or No to determine if you need to head to the dentist.

_____ Do your gums regularly bleed after brushing? If they do, it's an early sign of gingivitis or inflammation of the gums—which can be an early sign of periodontitis.

_____ Are your gums red? Healthy gums are coral pink and hold teeth tight. Inflamed gums are red, and the teeth may be loose.

*continued*

____ Are your gums retreating? If your gums are receding, maybe even far enough to expose the roots of your teeth, the situation is serious and needs attention right away.

Another way to tell if your teeth need attention is pain—although different types of pain may or may not mean that a trip to the dentist is warranted. Answer these questions Yes or No. Do you have:

____ 1. Momentary pain after eating hot or cold foods?
____ 2. Sharp pain when biting food?
____ 3. Lingering pain after eating hot or cold foods?
____ 4. Constant, severe pain and pressure, swollen gums and sensitivity to touch?
____ 5. Dull ache and pressure in the upper teeth and jaw?
____ 6. Chronic pain in your head, neck and/or ear?

## INTERPRETING YOUR ANSWERS

1. Generally speaking, momentary sensitivity of the gums is not a sign of a serious problem. It may be due to a loose filling or some gum recession that's exposing nerve-rich root surfaces. Try using a softer brush. And brush up and down instead of sideways, which can wear away exposed root surfaces. Also, try using one of the toothpastes for sensitive teeth.
2. Time to see the dentist. This could be a loose filling, a cracked tooth or a damaged pulp. Serious stuff, so act fast if you want to save the tooth.
3. This could be serious. You may have a deep cavity or physical damage to one or more teeth. See your dentist or endodontist right away.
4. This may be an abscess. See your dentist or endodontist as soon as possible. Meanwhile, take an over-the-counter pain reliever.
5. This could be a sinus headache, or it could be caused by bruxism (teeth grinding). Your dentist can help with the bruxism.
6. This could be caused by pulp-damaged teeth or other dental problems. See your dentist.

# 49

# THIN HAIR

Magic Tricks for Thicker Locks

If you find yourself lingering a bit longer at the bathroom mirror these days, peering at your scalp, alternately worrying and telling yourself that you've got as much hair as ever, stop fussing and fretting. Thinning hair is not hopeless: You can do plenty to make your hair look fuller, if not halt the hair loss.

Generally, men and women experience thinning hair for the same reason: androgenetic alopecia. This is just a fancy way of saying that certain hair follicles on the scalp are genetically programmed, not to die, but to slow down. Triggered by hormonal changes, the normal cycle of growth and rest becomes lopsided in the resting phase. So the scalp hairs never grow very long or very thick.

That's where the similarity between men's hair and women's ends. For while men frequently go completely bald from hereditary hair loss, women rarely do. Men and women lose hair in other, more noticeably different ways, says Allan L. Kayne, M.D., clinical assistant professor of medicine at the University of Washington and staff dermatologist at the Virginia Mason Clinic, both in Seattle. "The pattern looks different in women. They don't get thinning around the temples, but hair *does* thin out over the central scalp toward the front. Normally, a little band of hair at the front, right above the forehead, remains intact," he says.

The bottom line is that thinning hair does not have to affect the way you look and feel. There's a lot you can do to retain fullness and beauty by working *with* your hair, not against it. Here are some tips on doing just that.

### Maybe the Cause Is Temporary

While most thinning is hereditary, there are also preventable and treatable medical conditions that cause hair loss. Your doctor is the best person to help you figure out if one of them is at the root of your problem.

"Both men and women should be aware of other medical problems that can influence hair," says Arthur P. Bertolino, M.D., Ph.D., associate clinical professor of dermatology and director of the Hair Consultation Unit at New York University Medical Center. "More than one cause could be responsible for your hair loss: systemic illness, stress, high fever, underactive thyroid, stopping birth control pills, giving birth and a variety of drugs. If an underlying cause is discovered, that can be treated. Or perhaps time is all that's needed, like in the case of hair loss after pregnancy. The hair will grow back within 6 to 18 months," he says.

---

## TRY TO UNWIND

There's a chance that your thinning hair is linked to your lifestyle. Hair loss in women has increased 45 percent in the past 25 years, and the cause may be elevated hormone levels caused by stress, according to Douglas D. Altchek, M.D., assistant clinical professor of dermatology at Mount Sinai School of Medicine in New York.

"Stress generates aggression, and aggression causes an increase of the male hormone testosterone in women," says Dr. Altchek. "The testosterone reaches the hair root and causes shrinkage of the hair shaft. The result could be a loss of hair."

---

It's a good idea to ask your doctor if your hair loss could be caused by any of these conditions. And if your hair is shedding in clumps or handfuls, or you have a rash or sores on your scalp, head for the doctor. "Shedding means you might have handfuls of hair in your comb or brush or shower," says Dr. Kayne. "Shedding is not a symptom of androgenetic alopecia. Something else may be going on, such as an infection."

## BEEF UP YOUR DIET

Hair volume can be related to how well you're eating, says Dr. Kayne. "The body has a clever way of knowing which body structures are not so important, like the hair on your head," he says. "If nutritional intake is limited, hair suffers before the vital organs. So when you go on a severe fad diet—concentrating only on fruit, for example—you may experience hair loss." The loss is temporary, he points out, and will reverse itself once you start eating a balanced diet.

Since hair is largely made of protein, dietary protein is the most important nutrient for your hair. Anything that severely limits your daily protein intake (such as crash dieting) will threaten your hair, according to Dr. Kayne.

Getting enough of the mineral zinc is also important. One study found that when a zinc deficiency was corrected by supplementation, hair loss not only stopped but was reversed. You can find zinc in whole-grain products, seafood, meat and wheat bran and germ, or in most multi-vitamin-and-mineral supplements.

## WORK WITH YOUR HAIR

If your diet's just fine and your locks are still thinning, there are plenty of easy ways to make your hair *look* fuller. Here's how.

**Try a new 'do.** "Most women who experience hereditary thinning can mask it successfully just by selecting a new hairstyle," says Vera Price, M.D., clinical professor of dermatology at the University of California, San Francisco. "For example, you could comb your hair over the thinning section, or perm it for a shorter, fluffier appearance."

"Ask your hairstylist what looks good on your face," advised Dr. Kayne. "Most stylists agree that the best cuts for thin hair are the shorter styles, which help mask the fact that some areas have less hair. You don't want to part it where the thinning is obvious. If you're going to part it at all, part it off to the side, not down the middle, where it's likely to be thinnest. And using a style such as a ponytail or braids or cornrows—anything where you're gathering it up—is bad. Don't use clips or barrettes."

**Pump it up.** Hair-thickening agents, such as gels and mousses, may measurably improve the fullness of your hair, according to Dr. Bertolino. "These products don't change the hair in any way but merely add bulk to the hair shaft," he says.

Try using a styling spritz to add volume. This is simple: Spritz your hair, then finger-comb it—or use a pick—to lift it off the scalp and add volume as it dries.

**Don't weigh it down.** The same wonderful chemicals that add bulk also add weight, which can flatten your hair, so don't allow these chemicals to accumulate. Remember also that conditioners are formulated to cling to the hair shaft and not rinse away. With repeated use, this film can build up and attract dirt, leaving your hair looking limp.

To avoid flat, overly conditioned hair, lather up with a non-conditioning shampoo once or twice a week. Look for brands formulated specifically for people who use mousses, hair sprays and other conditioning chemicals.

**Wash as often as needed.** Don't think that by washing your hair less, you're preventing it from falling out. Unless you scrub too aggressively, washing your hair will not accelerate hair loss. But not sudsing up may allow dust, dirt and your hair's natural oils to accumulate and weigh it down, thus making it appear thinner. Shampooing daily will avoid this problem.

**Try a perm or new color.** "You can also make thin hair appear thicker by perming or coloring it," says Dr. Bertolino. A perm bends the hair at the roots so it takes up more space than untreated hair, he explains, and altering hair color so it contracts less with the scalp color can also help conceal the fact that your hair is thinning.

**Be kind to your tresses.** "If you're concerned about thin hair, don't damage the hair you've got," says Dr. Kayne. "If you use a curling iron, hot comb, rollers, hot oil, hot blow dryer—anything that can mechanically damage hair—you're going to break hair off and make it look even thinner. Even excessive perms will damage and further thin your hair."

**Call in reinforcements.** For severely thinning hair or baldness, you may decide to go a step further and ask your doctor about hair transplants or drug treatments to stop hair loss. (See chapter 39.)

## ANTI-AGING CHECKUP
# TAKE STOCK OF YOUR LOCKS

Okay, maybe you think you've been noticing more hairs on your comb—but you're not sure, really. . . . And it *is* pretty difficult to get a good look at the top of your own head. "How thick or thin your hair looks is a very subjective judgment," says Marta Petersen, M.D., assistant professor of medicine at the University of Utah in Salt Lake City. "You can lose 50 percent of your total hair before it becomes obvious."

How can you tell if your hair is thin? Respond Yes or No to the following statements.

_____ 1. If I hold a handful of my hair up to the light, I can see through it.

_____ 2. I can see more of my scalp when there is a bright light over my head.

_____ 3. When I pull my hair back, the ponytail is less than an inch thick at the middle.

_____ 4. When I part my hair, the part line appears wider than it once did.

_____ 5. When I pull my hair back into a ponytail, I don't have as much fullness as I once did.

_____ 6. If I take a handful of scalp hairs and gently pull on them before shampooing, I can pull out more than 6 to 12.

### INTERPRETING YOUR ANSWERS

If you answered *any* of these questions Yes, your hair is definitely thin—although it doesn't necessarily mean that it's thinning.

A Yes to questions 1, 2 or 3 means your hair is thin, but it could be naturally that way. A Yes to question 4 alerts you that your hair is getting progressively thinner. Questions 5 and 6 are the best measures of whether or not your hair is thinning, according to Arthur P. Bertolino, M.D., Ph.D., associate clinical professor of dermatology and director of the Hair Consultation Unit at New York University Medical Center.

# 50

# WRINKLES

### New Hope for Crinkles and Creases

**Now** you can add wrinkles to the list of things that you don't have to learn to live with. Sooner or later everyone gets some lines, but you can minimize the damage with simple preventive measures. And not only can you head off much of what you might have thought were inevitable signs of aging, but— thanks to some newly developed treatments—you can undo at least some damage that has already occurred. Follow this pre-emptive strategy, and you can take months or even years off your appearance.

### SUNSCREEN: YOUR NUMBER ONE WEAPON

One of the easiest, most effective and inexpensive ways to help prevent wrinkles is by faithfully using sunscreen. "The number one contributor to how old your skin looks is ultraviolet sun damage," says Ronald Sherman, M.D., senior clinical instructor in dermatology at Mount Sinai Medical Center in New York. "It destroys the ability of your skin to renew itself at peak capacity." Sun exposure is what deepens your smile lines and frown lines and brings out crow's feet.

"Sun damage is responsible for most of what we think of as skin's aging, such as wrinkles as well as discoloration, growths and skin cancers," says Jeffrey H. Binstock, M.D., assistant clinical professor of dermatologic surgery at the University of California, San Francisco. "The bottom line is that if you're going to be outside in the sun, even for a short period of time, you should wear a sunscreen."

For maximum protection, make sure your sunscreen protects against both the UVA (ultraviolet A) and UVB (ultraviolet B) parts of the ultraviolet-light spectrum, suggests dermatologist O. J. Rustad, M.D., in *The Physician and Sports Medicine*. UVB is more likely to tan, burn and put you at higher risk for skin cancer. It is more intense in the summer and peaks during late morning and early afternoon (11:00 A.M. to 3:00 P.M. during daylight savings time). UVA is strong all year long, though it is less likely to produce a sunburn or skin cancer. UVA worsens the damaging effects of UVB, however. Plus, it penetrates deeper and destroys the elastin, spongy tissue that keeps your skin soft, smooth and pliable. Most wrinkling seems to be caused by UVA exposure, according to Dr. Rustad.

Using sunscreen has an added benefit: By blocking further sun damage and allowing repair, prior sun damage may be reversed as new "virgin" cells take the place of older, sun-beaten cells.

### MORE WRINKLE-FIGHTING TACTICS

Applying sunscreen isn't the *only* thing you can do to help prevent your skin from wrinkling. Here are more helpful measures.

**Dab on moisturizer with sunscreen.** In a study at the University of California, Irvine, a treatment that combined a sunscreen and moisturizer resulted in improvement in brown spots, wrinkling and skin roughness in almost half the users. "Using the two together may turn out to be the best treatment of all," says Edward Jeffes, M.D., Ph.D., associate professor in the department of dermatology at the University of California, Irvine, and assistant chief of dermatology at Long Beach Veterans Administration Medical Center.

**Nix cigarettes.** Smokers are nearly five times more likely than nonsmokers to show excessive skin wrinkling. Smoking may hasten wrinkling by damaging collagen, the fibrous protein in skin that keeps it from drooping and sagging, according to Donald P. Kadunce, M.D., a dermatologist in private practice in Salt Lake City. "Smoke activates certain enzymes that destroy certain tissues in the lungs," says Dr. Kadunce. "It may do the same to the outside—harming the collagen and elastin in the skin." The result is a distinctly sallow complexion and cobblestone appearance, with a network of fine lines over the cheeks.

**Put on a Mona Lisa smile.** The less you contort your face, the better. A bland face minimizes expression lines—crow's-feet and so forth. But, short of maintaining a stone face, you may prevent furrows by not squinting, furrowing your brow or making other exaggerated facial expressions. The problem is, most people don't even know they are contorting their facial muscles. Try this: Place a mirror next to the telephone, and watch yourself the next time you're talking on the phone. You may be surprised to notice that you move your face a lot more than you thought. No one wants a face devoid of expression, but you can help prevent frown lines just by learning to relax your forehead.

**Wear shades.** The delicacy of the skin around the eyes makes it a prime target for the crinkly lines that are an early sign of photo-aged skin, and squinting worsens the lines. Sunglasses with lenses that block ultraviolet light will not only reduce glare and squinting but also protect the area from further sun damage.

**Sleep on your back.** If you're on your side, with your face scrunched between your arm and your pillow, you will reinforce any wrinkle lines you already have. Sleeping on your back is the best position for a youthful-looking, unlined face, according to Gary D. Monheit, M.D., associate professor of dermatology at the University of Alabama School of Medicine in Birmingham. "Sleep lines show up as a deepening of existing forehead lines and a crease on the side of the cheek," he says. To avoid this accordion look, change your sleep position.

## Nonsurgical Wrinkle Treatments

What if your face is already lined, and you long for a return to a smooth visage? Some topical medications can help remove your wrinkles. Here's the lowdown.

**Ask about tretinoin.** Tretinoin is a vitamin A derivative, originally developed as an anti-acne medication, that's been found to be an effective wrinkle eraser. In a study at the University of California, Irvine, the drug—which is applied topically—smoothed out sun-induced wrinkling and skin roughness in middle-aged people with moderately damaged skin. "It had already been shown to be effective in older people with severe damage," notes Dr. Jeffes.

Will it work on your wrinkles? "Our studies clearly show that people notice an improvement, especially in eliminating the fine lines around the eyes and softening coarse wrinkles on the upper portion of the face," says dermatologist Rodney Basler, M.D., assistant professor of internal medicine at the University of Nebraska Medical Center in Omaha, who is conducting clinical studies on the drug.

Tretinoin's effectiveness varies with each individual. Some people notice an improvement in the quality of their skin more than a disappearance of wrinkles. Also, some facial lines are too deep for tretinoin to reduce much. Experts recommend it be used regularly for 18 months to see the optimum effect, although improvement may be seen in 4 months.

**New-wave fruit acids.** Alpha-hydroxy acids (AHAs) are derivatives of certain fruits and other natural plant substances that can help lessen wrinkles—without the irritation that tretinoin can cause. "AHAs work much like tretinoin to reverse signs of aging," says James Leyden, M.D., professor of dermatology at the University of Pennsylvania in Philadelphia.

As skin ages, the epidermis shrinks, and there's a decrease in dermal glycosaminoglycans, compounds that are necessary to keep skin lubricated. Dr. Leyden's work with buffered ammonium lactate, a form of AHA, showed a significant increase in epidermal thickness and glycosaminoglycans.

In another study, 90 percent of the people using ammonium lactate showed slight or moderate improvement in their sun-damaged skin after 16 weeks, including improvements in both fine and coarse wrinkling, roughness, slackness and leatheriness.

At the strength used in these studies, AHA is available by prescription only, so check with your dermatologist. (Over-the-counter versions don't seem to work quite as well, say some sources.)

**Peel away the years.** In a chemical peel, various chemicals are applied to the skin, producing what doctors refer to as controlled wounding. (It looks like a very bad sunburn.) "The skin reacts by sloughing off several layers of skin cells and then regenerating new skin, which not only looks better but is also less prone to skin cancer," says Harold J. Brody, M.D., clinical associate professor of dermatology at Emory University School of Medicine in Atlanta.

Although a chemical peel is usually an outpatient procedure (done in a doctor's office), it disturbs enough tissue to be considered surgery and, like all surgery, involves certain risks. People with a family history of scarring or who take certain medications are advised against this procedure—which should *always* be performed by an experienced physician.

**Look into dermabrasion.** Dermabrasion removes damaged skin layers and can give excellent results, says Dr. Monheit. Wrinkled and damaged skin is removed with a special rotating wire brush or sanding instrument, leaving the skin temporarily somewhat raw. Normally used mainly for acne scars, dermabrasion can also be used for small wrinkles caused by sun damage. Though results last for years, the skin takes weeks to heal and may be scarred. You'll need to discuss the pros and cons of this treatment with your dermatologist. And don't schedule it right before your next class reunion or important business trip—you'll look worse before you look better.

**Fill in wrinkles with collagen.** For wrinkle lines that are more crevice than cobweb, especially when the rest of your skin tone is good and lines are isolated, many doctors apply one of a variety of substances—sort of like Spackle compound for your epidermis. The most commonly used filler material is injectable bovine collagen, a fibrous protein naturally present in skin that keeps it from sagging and drooping.

"The doctor will inject the collagen directly into the wrinkle until it's raised beyond the skin surface and forms a little lump," explains Dr. Monheit. "The lump may stay red for 12 to 24 hours, but when it fades, the skin surface is smooth."

Collagen injections are not a permanent cure. Over the course of time, your body absorbs the injected collage, and the wrinkle reappears.

**Plump them up with newer materials.** One new filler is

Fibrel, a gelatin-based implant that's mixed with the patient's own blood serum and injected. According to Dr. Monheit, Fibrel not only lasts longer than collagen—five years for some people—but causes fewer allergic reactions. This procedure, however, has more steps, requires more time and is more painful.

Another new technique is microlipoinjection, or fat transfer. This involves extracting a tiny amount of fat from one area of the body and using it to fill in another—usually the face and hands. Unfortunately, the fat cells don't seem to last very long in their new home. Sometimes they don't "take," or wrinkles reappear within several months.

One last word: Cosmetic surgery and other medical procedures are serious business. Don't feel pressured into techniques unless you're sure they're right for you. Sometimes, the "wax museum" look isn't worth the risks. If you can accept that a certain amount of facial aging is okay, your self-esteem will not suffer.

## ANTI-AGING CHECKUP
# WRINKLE-FIGHTING STRATEGIES

If you're worrying about wrinkles, don't. (Worrying makes them worse.) Instead, look in the mirror and answer these questions Yes or No to decide where your wrinkles may be coming from and what you can do about them.

_____ 1. Do you have a suntan?
_____ 2. Do you have frown lines?
_____ 3. Do you have squint lines?
_____ 4. Do you have crow's feet?
_____ 5. Do you have a crease line on the side of the cheek?
_____ 6. Do you have fine lines around the eyes?
_____ 7. Do you have coarse wrinkles on the upper face?
_____ 8. Do you have sun-induced spots and moderate skin damage?
_____ 9. Do you have sagging skin around the eyes?
_____ 10. Do you have firm but sun-damaged skin?

### INTERPRETING YOUR ANSWERS

What you can do for the problems you answered Yes to:

1. You should be using a sunscreen. A tan is an indication that your skin has already been exposed to the sun enough to damage it.
2. Learn to relax your forehead.
3. Wear sunglasses, use sunscreen, and take care not to squint.
4. Stop smoking. If you don't smoke, try staying out of smoke-filled rooms.
5. This is a sleep line. Sleep on your back.
6. Ask your dermatologist about tretinoin, which may eliminate the lines.
7. Again, talk to your dermatologist about tretinoin.
8. Try a moisturizer-sunscreen combination first. If it doesn't help, consider tretinoin.
9. If bags are very pronounced, cosmetic eye surgery may be the only option. If not, try not to let them upset you.
10. If you're willing to undergo the discomfort, you might consider a chemical peel.

# PART III
## Thinking and Feeling Young

# 51

# CREATIVITY

The Elusive Trait That Keeps You Young

**Can** it be true? Can a trait associated with youth be the key to *staying* young, decade after decade? The answer is yes—for a number of reasons.

Creativity can be a big help at any stage in life, and it seems to have special benefits as we get older. Creative people are more flexible and more open to new experiences, whether in their community, workplace or travels. They are more independent, more appreciative of beauty, have broader interests and are more tolerant of situations that are not clear-cut.

Intuitive thought—the ability to let your mind drift, zigzagging from one idea to the next—is a vital component of creativity. That's why so many great ideas tend to pop into your brain while you're driving, showering or nodding off to sleep.

All this "irrational" thought actually comes in handy in some very practical ways. A Swedish study found that creative people are more flexible in dealing with anxiety-provoking situations. They are able to call upon the full mental energies of both their rational left and creative right brains to solve problems.

Creative people have been found to be more likely to adjust well to aging and even more likely to use humor and selflessness to aid in that adjustment. A study at the University of Nebraska in Lincoln found that creativity can help people grow through the aging process and find meaning in life. Many of the people in that study said that being creative enhanced their satisfaction in life.

It's clear that creativity is definitely something you want to cultivate as you get older.

## You Don't Have to Be a Genius to Be a Genius

Now comes even more good news. The young and the gifted do not have a monopoly on creativity. You can cultivate creativity in your own mental garden. Rembrandt's IQ is said to have been around 110—hardly enough to land him in the "gifted" class. But his lack of measurable genius didn't hold him back—and it shouldn't hold you back, either.

Don't assume that creativity wanes with the passage of time. *Au contraire*: In the University of Nebraska study, 60 percent of individuals interviewed felt they'd become more creative as they got older. Of the remaining 40 percent, half said they'd remained consistently creative throughout life.

So, *no excuses*. Here are some practical tips to pump up your brain power. Select the ones that suit you best, and practice them whenever you're faced with a complex problem or want to get the creative juices flowing as you tackle a hobby.

**Get rid of the static in your attic.** Don't let your creative instincts get drowned out by the noise from the rational "Mr Spock" part of your brain. Lynne Schwab, Ph.D., associate professor of education at the University of North Florida in Jacksonville, recommends a simple relaxation exercise to help you tune out the analytical and tune in to the creative and intuitive.

Sit with your feet flat on the floor and your eyes closed. Pay attention to your breathing. As you breathe in, imagine breathing in all the good things your body needs. As you breathe out, imagine letting out what you don't need. Now you are ready to think creatively, in peace.

**Think beyond reality.** You'll think more creatively if you take a slightly "crazy" look at any given situation or object. For example, the next time you look at an orange-juice can, tell yourself, "This could be a can—or it could be a pencil holder or a vase or a . . ." People taught to think this way are better at solving problems creatively, says Ellen Larger, author of *Mindfulness*.

**Don't forget how to play.** "Creativity most surely is a form of play," says George E. Vaillant, M.D., of the Dartmouth Medical School in Hanover, New Hampshire. It's a means of having fun, not just of resolving conflict. Dr. Vaillant, who conducted a long-term study of gifted women, concluded, "Retention of the capacity for play may be a critical ingredient for successful aging."

**The more ideas, the better.** When thinking creatively, "try to get as many ideas as you can," says Jim Shields, manager for innovation programs and products at the Center for Creative Leadership in Greensboro, North Carolina. The more ideas you generate, the higher the chances you will come up with a real winner.

**Suspend judgment.** Be careful not to critique or judge your ideas while you're generating them. You may not only slow down the pace but also stifle yourself. Jot down *all* your ideas, good or bad, then weed out the clunkers later.

**Stalk the wild ideas.** "I encourage people to think about ideas that might get them fired," quips Shields. That doesn't mean resorting to illegal, unethical or irresponsible notions. But allowing yourself to take some risks—at least hypothetically—may let you think of things you wouldn't ordinarily dare to imagine. You wouldn't want to live in a box. Why *think* in one?

**Take a walk—or a run.** You may cultivate your most creative thoughts somewhere around the block. Einstein did. In fact, he often became so wrapped up in creative thinking while on his walks that he got lost.

You don't have to be a genius physicist to get lost in creative walking. You don't have to get lost, either. A research psychologist at the Salt Lake City Veterans Administration Medical Center found that walking was just what a group of men needed to get their mental juices flowing. "Our fast-walking group significantly improved their mental abilities," says Robert Dustman, Ph.D. "The aerobic exercisers showed an improvement in short-term memory, had faster reaction times and were more creative than nonaerobic exercisers."

**ANTI-AGING CHECKUP**
# DISCOVER YOUR HIDDEN CREATIVITY

Are you creative? Marcia Yudkin thinks *everyone* is. "Creativity encompasses much more than the traditional arts," says the Boston writing and creativity consultant. "Almost everybody has something that they do differently from other people—and that's what creativity is." To reveal your latent creativity, Yudkin creatively put together this series of questions. Answer them Yes or No.

_____ Have you ever told a joke spontaneously?

_____ Have you ever told a joke differently from the way you heard it originally?

_____ Have you ever fulfilled a responsibility in a unique way?

_____ Have you ever made something—a lavishly decorated birthday cake, for instance—for sheer personal satisfaction?

_____ Have you ever applied a hobby at work (such as making a poster for a co-worker out on medical leave)?

_____ Have you ever solved a particularly thorny problem?

_____ Have you ever done something, no matter how simple or routine, in a way different from the way everyone else does it?

_____ Have you ever taken a chance by exploring a new jogging or walking route?

_____ Have you found a unique way to persuade your child or spouse to do the dishes?

_____ Have you ever made a vegetarian meal that pleased meat eaters?

_____ Have others admired your garden or indoor plants?

_____ Do you ever sing in the shower or in the car? Do you ever change the words?

_____ Do you know how to play a musical instrument?

*continued*

## INTERPRETING YOUR ANSWERS

The more Yes answers you give, the more likely you are to face life and its challenges with confidence and vigor. But even one Yes means you may be able to compose a symphony, paint a masterpiece or write a best-seller.

# 52

# DEPRESSION

### What to Do When You're Blue

**Like** happiness, a certain amount of sadness is natural. When we lose a loved one or a job, or experience a big disappointment, it's normal to feel sad. At mid-life, it's normal to feel a little sad when the kids go off to college or leave home to begin families of their own, normal to feel tired a little sooner at work and at play, normal to feel a twinge of regret every now and then when you think of dreams you had that may never be fulfilled.

But when that sadness doesn't go away . . . when fatigue colors your entire approach to life and saps your energy, when regret drains your enthusiasm, and maybe even haunts you with thoughts of ending it all . . . that's depression. And it's a problem you must do something about because depression can affect your life and health in many negative ways. If you're depressed, you won't be the same at work or at home. Your productivity can plummet, endangering your livelihood. Your family life can suffer. And in some circumstances, untreated depression can lead you to abandon all hope.

What's more, scientists are just beginning to uncover some surprising physical repercussions of unchecked depression. Depression weakens your immune system's ability to fight off disease. If you're depressed *and* you smoke, it's a deadly mix. Not only are depressed smokers less likely to quit, they're also more likely to develop cancer. Depression heightens your heart disease risk, too. A Finnish study showed that, all other risk factors being equal, depressed men had two to four times greater plaque buildup in their arteries than men who were not depressed.

The good news is that you can do something about depression. First, though, you've got to recognize that it's an illness, not a sign of character weakness. Once you take steps to do something about it, the odds are heavily in your favor. According to the National Institute of Mental Health, symptoms can be relieved in 80 percent of people with serious depression, usually in a matter of weeks. So you *can* climb out of depression—and here are some rungs on the ladder to a happier existence.

**Pile on the pasta.** When eaten by themselves, complex carbohydrates may lift you out of depression by boosting levels of the mood-stabilizing brain chemical serotonin, according to Judith Wurtman, Ph.D., a nutritional researcher at the Massachusetts Institute of Technology and author of *Managing Your Mind and Mood Through Food.* Dr. Wurtman recommends at least one meal each day that is high in complex carbohydrates, with little or no protein. Rice, potatoes and pasta are good choices.

**Hide the sugar and coffee.** Removing refined sugar and caffeine from your diet could be all you need to do to banish depression. A study at Texas A&M University prescribed and monitored this dietary maneuver on volunteers suffering from major depression for three weeks, then tested them. The group's scores on three standard tests for depression were significantly improved. Three months later, they were tested again, and their moods were better.

**B vitamins may brighten your day.** The B-complex vitamins play important roles in the metabolism of brain chemicals vital to clear thinking and a stable mood. And deficiencies of riboflavin, pyridoxine, cobalamin (vitamin $B_{12}$) and folate have been found in people suffering from major depression. In one English hospital, half of the depressed patients with diagnosed folate deficiency were given folate supplements. As a result, they showed significantly greater improvement in their symptoms than deficient patients not given folate. The severely ill patients were also receiving standard drug treatment for depression. In the doctors' opinion, correcting the folate deficiency enhanced the effect of the drugs.

**Stay up past your bedtime.** Don't laugh. Even a few hours of sleep deprivation can bring on rapid and dramatic reversal of depression. If you aren't suffering from sleep disturbance or insomnia, try staying up late one or two evenings to see if it improves your mood.

**Set your alarm clock for earlier.** Doctors don't know why sleep deprivation works or why depriving sleep at different times of the night seems to work better for different people. But if staying up later doesn't help, try getting up a couple of hours earlier instead. You don't have to *lose* any sleep; you can go to bed earlier to make up the difference.

**Distract yourself.** Fill your time with activities that will distract you from your negative thoughts. Depressed people who simply sit and ruminate about how sad they are or who try to figure out why they're so sad tend to stay depressed longer than people who plan positive changes and distractions. In studies with depressed people, moods improved among those who were given any distracting task, however meaningless or trivial. Those who were given tasks that tended to focus on their emotions became even more depressed.

**Start moving!** Exercise can improve your mood. Whether it's the increased blood flow to the brain, the release of endorphins and other feel-good hormones, the discharge of hostility, some reduction of emotional strain or all of the above, a regular program of aerobic exercise can improve your mood and raise your morale. Don't worry if you've been inactive much of your life. When inactive people finally do start exercising, their depression tends to lift.

**Talk to your doctor.** Your physician is the best person to see for a depression you can't shake. It might be caused by any of a number of physical problems—a side effect to a prescription drug, a thyroid problem, premenstrual syndrome, a hormone disturbance, diabetes, a quick-loss diet gone awry, sunlight deficiency or nutritional deficiencies. A comprehensive physical exam will reveal any of these problems. Or your depression may be severe enough to require antidepressant medication or some other medical treatment.

### Talk Yourself Out of a Funk

Friends may encourage you to "just pull yourself together," which is easier said than done. But there *are* mental steps you can take to lift yourself out of mild depression. For starters, you need to realize that those feelings of hopelessness and powerlessness may be very real to you but may not accurately reflect the way things are. Therapists who specialize in this form of self-talk call it cognitive therapy or cognitive restructuring. The idea is that you can truly make yourself miserable by thinking miserable or pessimistic thoughts—and vice versa: Think positive, happy thoughts and your mood will follow. Here is a step-by-step guide to help you get into the sunshine.

**Identify your depressing thoughts.** When you're feeling depressed, stop and listen closely to your own thoughts. Chances are you'll hear words like *never, hopeless, I wish, can't, haven't, should, shouldn't*—words that encourage doubt, guilt or pessimism or judge you harshly and put you down. These are powerful messages. Quite possibly, you were feeling just fine until one of these discouraging thoughts came along and sent your upbeat thoughts packing—and your mood into the cellar.

It doesn't have to be that way. Once you become aware that you're inflicting these thoughts on yourself, you can do something about them. So listen carefully and identify these destructive ideas. Write them down, if necessary, to get them out in the open.

**Just say "Stop" to discouraging words.** This is no time for a protracted debate. When you hear those discouraging, weakening inner messages, shout them down! You've got to be ruthless and tough. Don't give your damaging thoughts the chance to put you down.

At the same time, don't put yourself down, either. Don't judge yourself by saying things like "You're at it again!" or "Stop thinking that way, stupid!"

Although this sounds simple enough, it takes time and perseverance to get it right. It may help to ask yourself, "Is this thought helping me solve my problems?" If the answer is no, then your response should be "Stop!"

**Send yourself a positive "mental fax."** Once you've stopped the negative thought dead in its tracks, you need to replace it with something positive and uplifting. For example, suppose you find yourself pulled down by thoughts that nothing is going right in your life, that you've little to show for all those years. Once you've vanquished those thoughts, you must keep them from coming back by immediately thinking of something that is going *right* in your life. Concentrate on an accomplishment or an experience, however minor, that has given you pleasure and gives you pleasure to think about.

This technique will help to break down your problems—and your positive statements—into specific, workable units. For example, if you're haunted by thoughts such as "I'm a failure! I'll never succeed," replace them with specific plans for success, such as "I know what to do to make progress on this. What I don't know I can learn. I'm going to do my best, be patient and make progress."

**Chart a new course.** It's one thing to bash depressing thoughts as they come up and replace them with positive ones. But now it's time to look at your life from a broader, long-term perspective, get a firm grip on the wheel and steer your thoughts—and your actions—to the sunny side of the street. In other words, make plans to be happy and not depressed.

Write down the positive thoughts you have used to lift your mood. In other words, make a list of your strengths and assets, the fun and rewarding activities in your life, and your goals and plans for achieving them. Start to fill more and more of your time with these activities, working toward your goals and feeling satisfaction and pride in your strengths and achievements.

Keep this list handy, and refer to it when you feel the road taking a turn into the dark. It's your road map to the bright side.

## ANTI-AGING CHECKUP
# RATE YOUR MOOD

Depression is more than a passing blue mood, more than a twinge of sadness you feel on hearing an old love song. When you're depressed, your whole body can be depressed, not just your thoughts and moods. The effects of depression show up in the way you eat, the way you sleep, the way you work and even the way you play.

The following checklist from the National Institute of Mental Health will help you figure out if you're clinically depressed. Check the symptoms that have persisted for two weeks or longer.

\_\_\_\_ Persistent sad, anxious or empty mood

\_\_\_\_ Feelings of hopelessness and pessimism

\_\_\_\_ Loss of interest or pleasure in ordinary activities that you once enjoyed, such as a hobby or sex

\_\_\_\_ Fatigue, decreased energy, feeling "slowed down"

\_\_\_\_ Insomnia, early-morning awakening or oversleeping

\_\_\_\_ Eating disturbances: overeating and weight gain or loss of appetite and weight loss

\_\_\_\_ Difficulty concentrating, remembering and making decisions

\_\_\_\_ Feelings of guilt, worthlessness and helplessness

\_\_\_\_ Thoughts of death or suicide—or suicide attempts

\_\_\_\_ Restlessness and irritability

\_\_\_\_ Uncontrollable, excessive crying

\_\_\_\_ Chronic aches and pains that don't respond to treatment, such as headaches and digestive disorders

### INTERPRETING YOUR ANSWERS

If you have checked four or more of these symptoms or if any of them are interfering with your work or family life—or if you have suicidal thoughts—you should see a physician. A full diagnosis will include a complete physical checkup and a family history of health problems.

# 53

# HOSTILITY

Patience Is Good Medicine

**Think** about the smorgasbord of moods you experience during a routine day. Is there an undercurrent of irritation, annoyance and, yes, even outright hostility that flows just below the surface? Are you overcome by a surge of impatience when you're provoked by, say, a slow-moving line at the grocery store or a driver who cuts in front of you on the highway? If so, you may be raising your risk of a number of serious diseases. Hostility kills.

That's not to say you should *never* get angry. You'd have to be made of stone not to get annoyed or impatient occasionally. But anger is an immediate and temporary emotional arousal, while hostility is a negative attitude that doesn't go away. A hostile person feels angry more frequently because he or she expects others to behave badly, selfishly or otherwise unsatisfactorily.

"Cynicism compels the hostile person to constantly be on guard against the 'misbehavior' of others. The slightest negative provocation can then set off angry feelings and aggressive behavior," says Redford B. Williams, M.D., professor of psychiatry and director of the Behavioral Medicine Research Center at Duke University Medical Center in Durham, North Carolina, and coauthor (with his wife, Virginia Williams, Ph.D.) of *Anger Kills: Seventeen Strategies for Controlling the Hostility That Can Harm Your Health.*

The negative effects of a bad attitude aren't limited to your emotions. Hostility can raise your levels of total cholesterol, lower your level of beneficial HDL cholesterol and raise your blood level of dangerous fats called triglycerides. And statistics show that hostility doesn't exist in a vacuum—distrustful people are also more likely to smoke, drink too much alcohol, load up on caffeine and consume too much cholesterol or total fat (or overeat in general). Chronically frustrated and hostile folks frequently end up with high blood pressure and suffer from arthritis. Add it all up, and it's no wonder that hostile people run a great risk not only of heart disease but of dying of *all* causes.

## ATTITUDE ADJUSTMENT FOR THE CHRONICALLY ANNOYED

Can a hostile "leopard" change its psychological "spots"? Or are hostile souls doomed to let their hostility eat away at their health?

Luckily, hostility can be controlled—with some work. "Controlling hostility is not simple," says Dr. Williams. "It takes time and effort—but you can make progress. With practice, you can change your cynical perceptions, behave more kindly toward others, reduce the number of situations that arouse you to anger and rein in your anger before you lose control."

With that hopeful attitude in mind, here are some tips to help you cultivate a more trusting, less hostile soul.

**Stop hostility in its tracks.** "You can short-circuit your hostile thoughts by silently shouting 'Stop!' to yourself," says Dr. Williams. If you're alone, say it out loud. "You'll be surprised how well this simple strategy works to get rid of those everyday hostile thoughts, feelings and urges that haunt hostile people.

"It helps to have a pleasant thought in reserve, something you enjoy thinking about, like a favorite person or activity, to replace the hostile thought," he adds. If someone pulls in front of you in traffic, imagine something pleasant, like schussing on skis and slowing to navigate a mogul, for example.

**Be quiet and listen.** "Because they tend not to trust others, most hostile people are very self-involved," says Dr. Williams. "They feel they have only themselves to count on." As a

## ANTI-AGING CHECKUP
# ARE YOU A TRUSTING SOUL?

What's your hostility quotient? Are you inwardly hostile enough to damage your own health? This self-check will help you find out.

One caveat: "We're all tempted to choose the response we think we ought to pick," cautions Redford B. Williams, M.D., professor of psychiatry and director of the Behavioral Medicine Research Center at Duke University Medical Center in Durham, North Carolina, and coauthor (with his wife, Virginia Williams, Ph.D.) of *Anger Kills: Seventeen Strategies for Controlling the Hostility That Can Harm Your Health.* "Instead, answer as honestly and spontaneously as you can."

Choose only one response for each situation. Don't worry if neither response seems to fit—or if both do. This is normal. Just indicate the one that is more likely for you.

1. A really important job needs to be done.
____ a. I prefer to do it myself.
____ b. I am apt to call on my co-workers to help.
2. A teenager drives by my house with the stereo blaring heavy-metal or rap music.
____ a. I can feel my blood pressure start to rise.
____ b. I begin to understand why teenagers can't hear.
3. I see a very overweight person walking down the street.
____ a. I wonder why these people have so little self-control.
____ b. I think that he or she might have a metabolic defect or a psychological problem.
4. I am in the express checkout line at the supermarket. A sign reads, "No More Than 10 Items, Please," but things are moving slowly.
____ a. I glance ahead to see if anyone has more than ten items.
____ b. I pick up a magazine to pass the time.
5. I am stuck in a traffic jam.
____ a. I immediately start to feel irritated and annoyed.
____ b. I'm usually not particularly upset.

*continued*

6. Another driver cuts in front of me in traffic.

_____ a. I usually flash my lights or honk my horn.

_____ b. I stay farther behind such a driver.

7. I recall something that angered me previously.

_____ a. I feel angry all over again.

_____ b. The memory doesn't bother me nearly as much as the actual event did.

8. Someone is speaking to me very slowly.

_____ a. I am apt to finish his or her sentences.

_____ b. I am apt to listen until he or she finishes.

9. Someone is dominating the conversation at a party.

_____ a. I look for an opportunity to put him or her down.

_____ b. I soon move to another group.

**Total:** _____

## INTERPRETING YOUR ANSWERS

Give yourself 1 point for every (a.) answer, ) 0 for every (b.) answer. If you scored a total of 0 or 1, your hostility level is relatively low and not likely to jeopardize your health. A score of 2 or 3 is borderline. A score of 4 or higher means you should practice ways to control your hostility.

SOURCE: From *Anger Kills* by Redford B. Williams, M.D., and Virginia Williams, Ph. D. Copyright © 1993 by Redford B. Williams, M.D., and Virginia Williams. Reprinted by permission of Times Books, a division of Random House, Inc.

result, they seldom pay close attention to what anyone else is saying. "Listening is foolproof," says Dr. Williams. "Force yourself to keep your mouth shut, lean forward and look intently at the other person. It's like a meditation, and it can have the same kind of relaxing effect. You'll really hear and understand what the other person says, and the likelihood of an argument will diminish."

**Give folks a chance.** Hostile individuals seldom allow themselves to depend on others, even in the most trivial everyday matters. They (erroneously) assume that they alone can (and must) take charge of every situation at home, at work or in their travels. "Force yourself to give up control," says Dr. Williams. "You'll feel truly liberated from the burden of having to be in charge of every situation in your life."

**Take up community service.** To overcome the tendency to focus on themselves, hostile people need to direct their attention outward, in a selfless way. "Giving up some of your time to volunteer public service will reduce your isolation and connect you with others in a healthy way," says Dr. Williams. "Altruism may help you live longer." You'll enjoy the change—and it will do you good.

**Empathize.** Dr. Williams has found that when we are able to see a situation through the other person's eyes, we can short-circuit the cynical reactions before they generate the anger that is so harmful to our health and our relationships. "To be more empathic," he says, "don't automatically assume the other person's motives are evil. Instead, imagine scenarios in which his or her behavior would be acceptable."

**Practice good old-fashioned tolerance.** "Allow other people to have beliefs, practices and habits different from your own," recommends Dr. Williams. "When we're intolerant, we perceive others as misbehaving—so we get angry. Try to accept other people as they are, not as you would like them to be." (After all, chances are that somewhere along the line, others have had to give *you* some latitude, right?)

**Forgive and let go.** Even if you've been truly wronged, don't dwell on the hurt or relive the event in your mind. Let it go. "Acknowledge that the person did wrong you," says Dr. Williams, "but consciously choose to forgive him or her. Wipe out the debt. You don't have to forget it or fail to be on guard against it happening again, but just forgive this specific event."

**Tap into "buddy power."** "Have a confidant," suggests Dr. Williams. "It can be a spouse or a close friend, but you should feel able to rely on that person for emotional or physical help—and vice versa, of course. Deep friendships help us survive and bring out the best in us."

**Laugh at yourself.** Nobody's perfect: If others can make mistakes (and all too often, they do), so can you. Enjoying a good laugh at your own expense may be the best investment you ever make, according to Dr. Williams. "By seeing the humor in an unpleasant situation and laughing at yourself, you can force anger and the harmful physical effects that go with it from your mind and body," he says.

**Pretend today is your last.** Countless individuals who've come face-to-face with their own mortality report that afterward, they can more easily focus on what's important and what's not. "We give a 'last day' assignment in our workshops," says Dr. Williams, "and we have yet to hear anyone say they would spend their last day tidying up things at the office or settling an old grudge. It's possible to live every day with that kind of attitude, and it will reduce stress, anxiety and hostility." So instead of focusing your attention on petty annoyances, concentrate on the good you and others can do.

**Soothe with healing foods.** Consuming less cholesterol-laden food and improving your diet in other ways can help you improve your attitude, according to a study conducted by Sonja L. Connor, William E. Connor, M.D., and others at the State University of New York at Stony Brook and the Oregon Health Sciences University in Portland. In their study, people were assigned to one of four diets with varying amounts of fat. Those who consumed a diet with 30 percent or fewer of its calories from fat and high in complex carbohydrates were less hostile or depressed than people who ate a typical American diet with 37 percent of its calories from fat. Evidently, low-fat, high-carbohydrate fare improves psychological well-being and does arteries a favor.

# 54

# LEARNING

Be Your Own Best Teacher

**The** saying "You can't teach an old dog new tricks" may b
true for canines, but not for people. Our capacity to learn nev
things does not diminish as we get older. The mind remain
quite plastic and open, even eager, for new business. In fac
the learning "muscle," just like other muscles, gets stronge
the more we use it—regardless of age.

This isn't to say that getting older doesn't have *some* effec
on learning. "There are certain aspects of the ability to lear
that do seem to decline with age," says James Fozard, Ph.D.
associate director for the Baltimore Longitudinal Study o
Aging, National Institute on Aging (NIA), Gerontology Re
search Center, in Baltimore, Maryland. "In particular, olde
people appear to take longer to learn arbitrary things, like vo
cabulary or shopping lists. Seventy-year-olds require mor
time and study-test repetitions than 20-year-olds."

But it's possible to counteract some of these apparently di
minished abilities.

## Keep Your Mind Supple

Sometimes the only problem is lack of practice, says Dr
Fozard. "Learning is partly a skill, and it's very amenable t
training," he says. "Much of what's lost is probably lost from
disuse. Why would the healthy older people take more time t
learn? One explanation is that memorizing arbitrary lists i
simply not the kind of learning skill that we need much. Whe

do you have to learn these kinds of things most in your life? When you're a student. When you're older, the kind of learning you do doesn't depend much on that skill. But if you do need the skill, you can develop it."

Even the partial loss of brain cells that accompanies aging doesn't necessarily mean a loss in learning ability. The brain, if stimulated, can actually grow in other areas to make up for that loss, says Gene Cohen, M.D., Ph.D., director of the Washington, D.C., Center on Aging, and former acting director of the NIA, part of the National Institutes of Health in Bethesda, Maryland. "There is a body of research on animals that goes back 30 years showing that when animals are exposed to a more challenging or enriched environment—such as a more difficult maze or a bigger piece of cheese—some very interesting changes take place," says Dr. Cohen. Brain cells communicate via branching neurons called dendrites, and in these cases, *new* dendrites sprout. Also, aging doesn't stop these changes, he says.

Does the same growth take place in the human brain? While the evidence for that kind of plasticity comes mainly from animal studies, the growth may very well occur in people as well. "We infer from training and performance studies that the same thing does happen in humans," says Dr. Cohen. "Mental stimulation does enable the brain to maintain and even increase its capacity."

## TIPS TO IMPROVE LEARNING

Here are some suggestions to help you live and learn. Think of them as gardening tips, to make those dendrites sprout like never before.

**Move your body, raise your IQ.** Regular exercise will help keep you on your toes mentally, according to a study at Scripps College in Claremont, California. When highly active exercisers ages 55 to 91 were compared with a group the same age who did not exercise, the researchers found that the high-exercise group performed significantly better in all reasoning tests, in all reaction-time tests and two out of three memory tests.

Louis Clarkson-Smith, Ph.D., who conducted the research,

says, "I think this study strongly suggests that exercise is important in preserving our mental abilities as we get older." Some researchers speculate that the decline of mental and physical energy as we age is linked to a decline in our central nervous system's efficiency, which may be affected by circulation to the brain. So physical exercise, which is known to improve the efficiency of circulation, may help keep the cognitive skills fresh.

**Think of your life as a patchwork quilt.** "Challenge yourself in different ways," says Dr. Cohen. "To stay healthy, sharp and mentally responsive, you must exercise yourself mentally, physically and interpersonally." He recommends taking up a variety of different activities, some physically active and some not, some individual and some in groups. "This way, as you get older, if there is a change in your interests or physical capacity, you are not left without stimulating activities," he says. Some individual activities might include reading, model building, nature photography or walking. For group activities, you could join a book-discussion club, take up dancing or play a team sport.

**Follow your passion.** Challenge and stimulate your mind with activities you enjoy. For some folks, that's a daily crossword puzzle—which others may find a bore. "As long as you're interested in something and in touch with it, you're going to be stimulated by what's going on," says Dr. Fozard, who leads a Dixieland jazz band.

**Take your time.** Give yourself extra time to learn new things. "Under normal conditions, older people can learn and solve problems as well as younger people—just more slowly," says Stanley Coren, Ph.D., professor of psychology at the University of British Columbia in Vancouver. In one study, researchers found that older adults required more time to learn new skills but learned those skills as well as young people did.

**Test yourself.** You'll learn faster and better if you alternate between cycles of studying and testing yourself. "If you're helping your kids with their homework, how do you usually do it? You test them," says Dr. Fozard. "Then you help them work on the things they haven't learned yet. Then you test again. That's good advice at any age."

**Don't cram.** "Cramming is stressful and really doesn't

work for long-term learning," says psychologist Tony Buzan, author of *Use Both Sides of Your Brain* and coauthor of *The Mind Map: Radiant Thinking*. He says it's all right to work through an inspired burst of creativity, even if it lasts all night. But don't save all your studying for the night before a test, thinking you can force the information into your head.

**Use all your senses.** Hiding yourself away in a corner is not the best way to study for a test or prepare for a meeting. Instead, involve as many senses as you can. You'll learn better, for example, outside in the fresh air—where there are colors and smells and sounds—than you will in a cubicle in the library. While indoors, you can engage more senses by sitting in a different chair, working in a different room, decorating your office with bright colors or bringing in flowers or flower scents.

**Doodle as you take notes.** Who says that notes have to proceed in a straight line? According to Buzan, it's okay if your notes wind up looking more like pinwheels, trees, spider webs or a multicolored map of the solar system. That method of notetaking better mirrors the way most of us think, he says, and uses more of your brain's thinking and learning capacity.

**Let ideas simmer while you sleep.** A good night's sleep after soaking up new information may be crucial to lock it in that knowledge. A study at Trent University in Peterborough, Ontario, found that students who weren't allowed to sleep all night or who were awakened whenever they entered the deep phase of slumber called rapid eye movement (REM) sleep couldn't remember a complex logic game the next day. They could, however, remember a list of paired words—which suggests that sleep is more important for complex topics than it is for simple memorization skills.

According to Dr. Clarkson-Smith, learning loss can be caused by delayed sleep as well as lack of sleep. "If you stay out late on Friday night and then sleep in late Saturday morning and get your full complement of sleep, you tend to think you are all right," he says. "But we've found this not to be true. When you're on a schedule, your body expects to have REM sleep at a certain time. If you delay the onset of sleep, you miss the REM sleep your body is accustomed to, and you lose information." REM sleep, says Dr. Clarkson-Smith, appears crucial for digesting new information into long-term memory.

**Check your zinc and iron.** Deficiencies in these minerals aren't common, but if you are low in zinc and iron, some studies suggest that your ability to learn may be diminished. Don't take either of these minerals without checking with your doctor, however, as both can have troublesome side effects.

---

### ANTI-AGING CHECKUP
# FIND YOUR PEAK LEARNING TIME

Do you find yourself slumping in the afternoon, but raring to go in the evenings? Or perhaps you feel the most energetic in the mornings.

Each of us has certain times of the day or even certain days of the week when our memory functions best, says Eugene Raudsepp, Ph.D., president of Princeton Creative Research, and author of *Creative Growth Games* and other books about mental skills. "There is no rule. Some people work very well in the morning, some during the night." The time when you do your best work is usually only two or three hours long, so it's worthwhile to find that time and save your most challenging tasks for that period, he says.

To find your peak learning period, keep an hourly log for a few weeks. Every hour, jot down how you feel and whether you seem to be alert and if tasks are going well.

When you sit down with your log, scan it carefully. Ask yourself, "When is my energy level highest? When do I have the most physical and mental energy? When do I seem to do the best work? When do I feel most fully alive?" suggests Dr. Raudsepp. You'll likely find that during certain periods, you are consistently more alert and vigorous. These hours are the times when you should schedule learning tasks.

---

# 55

# LONELINESS

Tap the Power of Friendship

**Stunning** research has put new meaning into the phrase "make friends for life." Whereas togetherness was once thought of as something that made life richer and better—which isn't anything to brush off—we now know that friends and family connections can actually help us live longer. After tracking the lives of more than 1,300 people who had been diagnosed with heart disease for up to nine years, researchers at Duke University Medical Center in Durham, North Carolina, concluded that friendship is a powerful protective factor.

"We knew in exquisite detail how well their hearts functioned at the start of the study and, therefore, what their survival rates should have been," says Redford B. Williams, M.D., professor of psychiatry and director of Duke's Behavioral Medicine Research Center. "What we found was that those patients with neither a spouse nor a friend were three times more likely to die than those involved in a caring relationship."

This isn't the first time research has demonstrated that friendship can be good medicine. Scientists have long recognized that lonely or socially isolated people are less healthy and more likely to die. So powerful is "the loneliness factor" that it rivals the damaging effects of risk factors such as cigarette smoking, blood pressure, blood lipids, obesity and lack of physical fitness.

In a classic study in Alameda County, California, researchers followed nearly 7,000 people for nine years. They found that for every age-group there was a direct relationship between community or social ties and a person's chance of dying for any reason. People with the most social contacts were the least likely to die during the nine-year study; those who were the most isolated faced the greatest risk of dying. And the greater risk wasn't linked to traditional factors such as smoking, excess body weight and lack of exercise.

Other studies have confirmed these results: Socially isolated people, whether healthy or suffering from heart disease, are three to five times more likely to die than people with the strongest intimate relationships.

Why? What is it about loneliness that whittles away at life? Why does friendship heal and protect?

Intimate relationships make people feel they are still valued in the eyes of their family and friends. In simple terms, what is provided is the security of being loved. The benefits of togetherness—having a partner or family—may be even more fundamental. Evidence from animal studies demonstrates that it may be the mere *presence* of familiar organisms and the relative frequency of contact with them that makes the difference between health and disease and life and death.

## CULTIVATE TOGETHERNESS

If you feel lonely sometimes, you're not alone. According to a Gallup poll, one-third of Americans feel lonely. Perhaps you're among them. Maybe that new job turned out to be too far away to maintain your friendships, and you now find yourself in a new place with a great job and no social life. Maybe you feel you're just too busy to put in the time and energy to make and keep friends. Maybe you're a "golf widow" and you want to spend those lonely Saturday afternoons with other people. Here are some tips to help you increase your own frequency of contact with people.

**Strike up a conversation with an acquaintance or two.** Often the best potential friends are the people around you. "There may be people with whom you now have a very casual relationship who could develop into good friends," says Carolyn Cutrona, Ph.D., clinical psychologist and professor of psychology at Iowa State University in Ames. "Maybe there's someone you see every day who has a desk in the next office. You can ask that person to coffee. Maybe it's someone with whom you're already having coffee or lunch regularly, or someone you're playing tennis with every now and then. The idea is to go one step further, to see if you can get to know the person better."

**Join a group you like.** To make new friends, join a church, club, interest group or support group. "People are always surprised at the number of groups and clubs you can join, if you bother to look," says Dr. Cutrona. "If none that you find interest you, maybe you should make the effort to develop new interests."

"Newcomers clubs, churches, hiking clubs, special-interest groups—they all work to help you make friends," says Robert S. Weiss, Ph.D., director of the work and family research unit at the University of Massachusetts-Boston. "It's important that you find the activity meaningful. Then ask yourself if you're willing to get engaged in a community that is organized around that activity."

**Look up a long-lost friend.** "Call a friend you haven't seen for a long time," suggests Dr. Cutrona. "We don't have to satisfy our loneliness needs in person all the time. Maybe there are people in other places who are meaningful to you that you just haven't talked to in a while."

**Become a student again.** "Sign up for a class at a local college, university or recreation center," says Dr. Cutrona. "These are great places to make new friends. Many institutions even have residency programs where they provide dormitories for participants and also plan social activities in addition to the academic courses."

**For a "helper's high," volunteer.** Getting involved in something bigger than yourself is an excellent way to make friends. "Sign up to do volunteer work at a hospital, library, homeless shelter, soup kitchen or nursery school," says Dr. Cutrona. "Helping somebody else can provide a real lift. So can volunteering for a political campaign."

**Adopt a four-legged friend.** Whoever said "a dog is man's best friend" knew what he was talking about. Intriguing research has demonstrated that a pet dog can be an even better stress buster than a human friend in certain situations. Researchers measured the stress response in women performing a difficult task in the presence of their best female friend, their dog and alone. The friend tended to make the women show more stress than if they worked at the task alone. However, the women showed little or no stress when their dogs were with them.

Researchers theorize that the pets evoked more positive feelings than the best friends and helped the women adapt to stress. But dogs, of course, aren't the only comforting pets— and they don't suit everyone's lifestyle. You may prefer the company of a cat, a rabbit or another animal.

### THE ART OF MAKING FRIENDS

Okay, so you've joined three clubs and worn out a pair of walking shoes and still no new friends. Don't despair. Maybe you need to go beyond that. Making friends can be easier if you follow a few simple rules.

**Practice making small talk.** Don't be afraid to talk about the mundane, like cars, sports, children, family—or the boss. "You don't have to open a conversation with something earth-shaking," says Dr. Cutrona. "Everybody talks about the weather. They do it all the time because it's something we all share. Everybody's kind of comfortable with it."

**Hang in there.** If you do the same things with the same people enough times, you will begin to develop friendships. "Find people who are more or less like you, and hang around with them," says Dr. Weiss. "Eventually, you'll be accepted and you'll make friends.

**Show genuine interest.** The secret here is to steer a casual relationship into slightly deeper waters by exchanging a bit more information. "Find out about the other person's concerns," says Dr. Cutrona. "Show genuine interest in what's going on in his or her life. Pay attention to what she says, and remember to ask about things she's told you. If you know her daughter was coming to see her, ask how the visit is going. Make a point of remembering what's going so you can

## ANTI-AGING CHECKUP
# HOW GOOD ARE YOU AT MAKING FRIENDS?

Answer the following questions Yes or No.

\_\_\_\_ 1. Do you find it easy to talk to people in the checkout line?

\_\_\_\_ 2. Do you feel relaxed talking to people you've met for the first time?

\_\_\_\_ 3. Do you smile at people when they hold the door for you?

\_\_\_\_ 4. Do you look at people when they're talking to you?

\_\_\_\_ 5. Do you know the names of more than half of the people you see every day, either at work or in your neighborhood?

\_\_\_\_ 6. Are you able to chat about the weather and other mundane things?

\_\_\_\_ 7. Do you feel comfortable asking a colleague or casual acquaintance to go for coffee?

\_\_\_\_ 8. Do you feel comfortable when someone shares personal information with you?

\_\_\_\_ 9. Are you a good listener?

\_\_\_\_ 10. Do you show appreciation when people do things for you?

\_\_\_\_ 11. Do you share your innermost secrets and feelings with ease with people you've just met?

\_\_\_\_ 12. Do you find the tips in this chapter scary?

## INTERPRETING YOUR ANSWERS

For the first ten questions, the more Yes answers, the better you are at making friends. However, if you answered number 11 Yes, the reverse is true. According to Carolyn Cutrona, Ph.D., clinical psychologist and professor of psychology at Iowa State University in Ames, "disclosing too much too soon is a characteristic of lonely people."

And for the folks who answered Yes to number 12? If you find these tips too scary to attempt, it might be a good idea to see a counselor who can give you some specific help on how to approach your problem of loneliness, suggests Dr. Cutrona.

refer to it in conversation. Maybe the other person will reciprocate, and the relationship can deepen into something more."

**Don't be too friendly too soon.** "Timing is important," says Dr. Cutrona. "Be careful you don't dump your most intimate secrets too soon. Take your time, and be patient. Friendship doesn't develop overnight. That's why it's best to express interest in the other person first and let that develop for a while. Take it slow, and if it doesn't seem to be going anywhere with one person, try somebody else."

# 56

# MEMORY

How to Remember Almost Everything

**Here's** a fact you may *want* to forget: Until lately, researchers have claimed that for every ten years an adult ages, his or her memory capacity declines 6 to 8 percent. Though the experts say this is normal, it's no comfort to think that significant pieces of mental luggage may be jarred loose and left behind as we accelerate farther down the bumpy road of life.

More recently, though, evidence suggests that in some ways our memory actually improves as we get older. According to gerontologists at the University of Oregon in Eugene, our memory's ability to adapt to the demands of the real world may actually improve as we get older. That's what they discovered when they tested the recall ability of a group of women age 70 against that of a group in their 20s or younger. Rather than ask the adults to memorize and recite random numbers, the researchers asked them to recall more meaningful information. The participants read a children's fable, then retold the tale to a young, attentive child. The older women respun the tale with less repetition and excess verbal baggage, while expressing the story more clearly and fluently than the younger women.

"We hoped they might do as well as the younger women, but when they actually did better, we were amazed," says Cynthia Adams, Ph.D., assistant professor of gerontology at the University of Oregon. "When these older women told their tale, they challenged the stereotype of age-related memory decline. It may be that as we grow older, we improve our ability to home in on the important themes found in information."

Nevertheless, we all know that certain things just seem to get bumped loose every now and then. Maybe we forget where we put down the car keys . . . or that letter from the IRS. And haven't we all had that embarrassing experience where we can't remember the name of a person we met five minutes ago—but can recall the words of a favorite song we knew 25 years ago? And when did the kids say you were supposed to pick them up? Was it at 6:00 or 6:30 P.M.?

To keep your brain revving at top speed, all you may need is better fuel.

**Don't forget your memory minerals.** "Certain nutrients may play an important role in our everyday behavior, though we don't know exactly how," says James Penland, Ph.D., research psychologist at the U.S. Department of Agriculture's Human Nutrition Research Center in Grand Forks, North Dakota. Several studies have found that low dietary and blood levels of iron, zinc and boron can compromise memory function.

In a pilot study, 34 young women with low blood levels of zinc and iron were given supplements to bring them up to par. After eight weeks, the women who took iron and zinc showed significant improvements in tests of short-term memory and attention over the women who didn't get the minerals.

In another study, researchers measured the effect of low zinc intakes on memory functions in 14 young, healthy men. They found that after low-zinc diets, the men performed worse on tests requiring short-term memory, spatial skills and attention than when they received a diet with about 10 milligrams of zinc daily. They also took *longer* to perform the tasks when consuming a low-zinc diet.

Deficiencies of these minerals are rare, but if your memory is flagging, ask your doctor if you may be low. Or boost your intake by eating more mineral-rich foods. Boron is in noncitrus fruits, legumes and cruciferous vegetables such as broccoli, cabbage and cauliflower. Good sources of zinc include whole-grain products, seafood and meat, and iron abounds in meat, poultry and fish. Don't, however, take iron or zinc supplements without checking with your doctor, as both can have serious side effects.

**Keep your noodle nimble with B vitamins.** Researchers checked brain function and nutrition status in 28 healthy people over the age of 60. Those with adequate levels of the B vitamin riboflavin had better memory performance, while those with adequate carotene levels were more agile on tests of cognitive (thinking) ability. People with high-iron status had brain-activity levels (measured by an EEG, an electroencephalogram) similar to young folks in their 20s and 30s—a healthy sign, according to the researchers. Those low on thiamine showed some impairment of brain activity. "It may be that nutrients are as vital for the brain as they are for the rest of the body," says Dr. Penland.

You don't need to go overboard in the name of mental gymnastics, though. You can achieve the same nutrient levels as the more successful study participants just by meeting the Recommended Dietary Allowances, says Dr. Penland. A balanced diet that relies on lean meats, fish, fruits, vegetables and grains can do the trick.

## SET THE STAGE FOR SUCCESS

The point to remember is this: Your memory is probably better than you think, and you can make it better still, regardless of your age. Here's how you can smooth out some of those bumps in memory lane.

**Hike up your memory function.** "By becoming actively involved in an exercise program, you may be able to help improve general short-term memory," says Richard Gordin, Ph.D., associate professor in the department of health, physical education and recreation at Utah State University in Logan. Dr. Gordin tested the effects of aerobic exercise on memory in three groups of people: those who exercised regularly, those who simply socialized and those who did nothing. "Compared with the other groups, the exercisers performed significantly better on general memory, especially verbal memory tests," says Dr. Gordin. He thinks that the aerobic exercise may have increased oxygen efficiency to the brain. "It may also spark an increase in glucose metabolism, which may play a role in increasing memory. This may be especially vital in recalling names, directions and telephone numbers or pairing a name with a face," he says.

**Forget your troubles.** Depression may make your trips down memory lane seem rougher than they really are. Researchers found that people rated their memories significantly poorer when they were depressed, despite the results of actual memory tests.

**A positive attitude helps.** "Bad attitude translates into bad memory," says Douglas J. Herrmann, Ph.D., researcher with the National Center for Health Statistics and author of *Super Memory*. "Your attitude has to be positive toward what you learn. If you're negative, in a bad mood or pessimistic, your memory is impaired. You don't pay as much attention. Then it's encoded in the brain as negative, and the mind usually chooses to forget unpleasant things."

**Take a deep breath.** Relaxation strengthens memory, says Dr. Herrmann. The idea is to balance your stress level. Whether you use yoga, music or chopping firewood, find a way to reduce stress. "If you find your memory failing during a test, my advice is to take a deep breath and hold it, then let it out slowly. This will relax you," he says.

**Memory works best in the comfort zone.** "Your memory works better if you're comfortable," says Dr. Herrmann. "If you have tight clothes on, have just eaten a heavy meal or have to go to the bathroom, you can't expect your memory to behave well."

### TRICKY TECHNIQUES TO HELP YOU REMEMBER

So you're well nourished, fit, relaxed and comfortable—and have a great attitude. But you *still* have trouble remembering things!

Don't sweat it. There are plenty of techniques you can utilize to help yourself learn and remember better. Here are a few.

**Use memory aids.** "Modern technology has come up with a lot of gadgets and tools to help us with memory. Take advantage of them," advises Dr. Herrmann. Automatic timers, telephones with memory speed-dialing, appointment books, things-to-do lists, pocket computers and notes stuck in prominent places can all serve as memory crutches. They'll help take the hassle out of your life and keep your mind clear for more important tasks.

**Give yourself time to digest material.** You can boost your ability to remember information if you don't cram. Instead, review material and allow some time to pass before going over it again. You'll remember more information by studying once a week for several weeks than you will by studying for several days.

**Sleep on it.** You've got that important presentation at work tomorrow, and it won't look good if you keep referring to your notes. How can you make sure you remember the material? Study it, and then hit the sack. According to Dr. Herrmann, if you go to sleep immediately after you learn something, you'll remember more than if you stay up and do something else before sleeping.

**Make a picture in your mind.** This memory-improvement strategy dates back to 300 B.C., according to Dr. Herrmann. A Greek poet was able to recall the names of every guest at a banquet by picturing them all in their places around each table. "The idea is to mentally put the images in a space that is familiar to you. It could be your home or anywhere. This strategy is very effective," Dr. Herrmann says.

**Form a sentence.** Repeat out loud something you need to remember, and make a sentence out of it: "I just met Sarah Smith, who comes from Des Moines," for example. "My research on techniques like this shows that they work," says Dr. Herrmann. "They force you to process the information and can increase recall by 300 percent."

**When in a bind, stall.** Often we feel rushed and pressured when we have to remember something—a name, a number, a date, an appointment. Dr. Herrmann says you don't have to be at the whim of the social situation. "You can control things so you have time to remember. Stall for time. You can do it quite deliberately. If you're at a meeting, say, "Let's get back to that point later.""

## ANTI-AGING CHECKUP
# HOW GOOD IS YOUR MEMORY?

The object of this test, from *Super Memory*, by Douglas Herrmann, Ph.D., is to come to grips with those areas in your life that are troublesome to your memory. "Everybody is good and bad at different things," says Dr. Herrmann, a researcher with the National Center for Health Statistics. "Even the person who thinks her memory is terrible is somewhat better at some things than at others."

Using numbers 1 (Always) to 7 (Never), estimate how often you remember these details of your daily life.

1—Always
2—Very often
3—Fairly often
4—About half the time
5—Now and then
6—Once in a while
7—Never

____ How often do you remember phone numbers without having to check?

____ How often are you able to recall the names of people you've recently met?

____ When you put something down and go to look for it a little while later, how often do you remember where you put it?

____ When you're in a restaurant and want to speak to your server, how often do you remember what he or she looks like?

____ How often do you remember what someone has just said to you?

____ When someone gives you directions to a destination, how often do you remember them on your way there?

____ When someone says he had told you something at an earlier time, how often can you remember what he said and when he said it?

____ After watching a movie or television show, how often are you able to remember the details?

*continued*

____When you have errands or several things to do, how often do you remember to do all the items on your mental list?

____Think of the times when you go to a room to get something. How often do you get to the room knowing why you're there?

____How often do you remember appointments?

____When performing an action that involves several steps, how often do you remember which step comes next?

## INTERPRETING YOUR ANSWERS

Most people, according to Dr. Herrmann, tend to answer with a 2 or 3—they remember things "very often" to "fairly often." The questions you answered with a number higher than 3 are most likely areas you need to work on.

# 57

# OPTIMISM

### The Benefits of a Positive Attitude

**Are** you an optimist or a pessimist? If someone says "Life after 40 is a bowl of cherries," do you think "Oh boy, I love cherries!" or "Gosh, I'm sure to break a tooth on one of the pits!"

Don't rush to answer. First, consider this: Optimists tend to do better in life. They may be happier, healthier and more successful. They may even live longer. And experts agree that for those people who accept the changes of aging with a positive, optimistic attitude—as a challenge rather than an inescapable turmoil—mid-life can be an exciting period of accelerated growth, renewal and fulfillment.

"There will always be people who are devastated by change," says Boston psychologist Joan Borysenko, Ph.D. "But more and more, we're finding people who view change as an opportunity rather than a threat." Call it what you want—optimism, looking on the bright side or viewing change as an opportunity—it works.

And a growing body of scientific literature reveals a link between pessimism and vulnerability to poor health. Most notably, Martin E. P. Seligman, Ph.D., author of *Learned Optimism*, and other researchers from the University of Pennsylvania in Philadelphia discovered that unrelenting pessimism can actually weaken the immune system.

In a classic study that demonstrates the health benefits of optimism, Dr. Seligman and his colleagues analyzed more than 35 years' worth of data on the health and psychological status of 200 men who graduated from Harvard University.

"The pessimistic men started to come down with the diseases of middle age earlier and more severely than the optimistic men," says Dr. Seligman.

Pessimists suffer in at least three ways, points out Dr. Seligman: "They are more vulnerable to depression, they achieve less than their talents would seem to predict, and their health is worse than an optimist's."

## THE WAY UP FROM DOWN

The important question is, can you change? Can you steer your attitude in a more optimistic direction?

You can, but it's not going to happen overnight. "It takes serious practice for two weeks or more to get the hang of optimism," says Dr. Seligman.

To become an optimist, you have to change how you view adversity. "Life inflicts the same setbacks on the optimist as on the pessimist," says Dr. Seligman. "The difference is that the pessimist believes bad things are permanent, pervasive and personal, while the optimist believes that bad things are temporary, specific and external."

The goal of the following steps is to get you to speak to yourself about your setbacks from a more encouraging, optimistic viewpoint. They are drawn from Dr. Seligman's clinical work helping pessimists to become more optimistic.

**Start with A, for Adversity.** Face it: Most days, life is a little like a Road Runner cartoon, full of all kinds of surprises, setbacks and obstacles. Next time you experience a setback, examine your thinking about it. Say you have a tiff with your spouse or a friend never seems to return your phone calls. How does that make you feel? Think about it carefully. Then proceed to the next step.

**Examine your beliefs.** How do you explain the adversity to yourself? If your spouse is short-tempered, do you decide it portends the end of your marriage, or do you just assume your spouse had a bad day? If your friend fails to call you, do you believe she's incredibly inconsiderate or assume she's just too busy? This is a crucial step, because negative assumptions become habitual beliefs—and they can have far-reaching consequences.

**Change the way you react.** You may think that your explanations of adversity are harmless. Quite the opposite is true, however. As Dr. Seligman says, "beliefs have a direct bearing on what we feel and what we do next. Beliefs make the difference between giving up or taking constructive action."

Let's say you believe your friend didn't call back because she's inconsiderate. The consequence of that might be that you feel depressed or angry at your friend. On the other hand, if you tell yourself that she's simply too busy right now, you wouldn't feel depressed or angry. More likely, you'd be understanding and receptive when you finally did talk to her again.

**Distract yourself.** When pessimistic thoughts enter your mind, try to think of something else. Dr. Seligman recommends ringing a bell, carrying a note card with the word STOP written in big red letters, wearing a rubber band on your wrist and snapping it to "snap out" of the negative thought or standing up and slapping the wall while shouting "Stop!" Then, while the negative thought is interrupted, replace it with another thought. Shift your concentration to something else. If negative thoughts persist, try writing about what's on your mind to ventilate your feelings, or simply schedule a later time for thinking about it.

**Argue with your pessimistic self.** "You can duck disturbing beliefs," says Dr. Seligman, "but a deeper, more lasting remedy is to give them an argument. If you dispute the pessimistic beliefs that come up during adversity, you can learn to be optimistic."

**Think temporary, not permanent.** If your original belief is that the cause of the problem is permanent, argue that the cause is really temporary and changeable. For example, if your boss asks you to redo an assignment, don't tell yourself you'll *never* be any good at reports—that would be permanent. Instead, tell yourself that you need more practice doing reports or that you didn't gather enough data or spend enough time on the report.

**Replace the pervasive with the specific.** If you flub a presentation at work, is it because you're terrible at public speaking or because you didn't prepare as well as usual? The first reason is pervasive and pessimistic, the second specific and optimistic.

**Don't take bad luck personally.** Believing you're somehow at fault for everything bad that happens is the mark of a pessimist. Optimists are better at shrugging off adversity. So if you explain that fight with your spouse by saying "I never do anything right," dispute it and replace it with something more like "He was just in a bad mood."

"Don't let pessimistic beliefs run your life," says Dr. Seligman. "Once you get in the habit of challenging them, your daily life will run much better, and you'll feel happier."

---

### ANTI-AGING CHECKUP
## ARE YOU AN OPTIMIST OR A PESSIMIST?

To use this quiz, adapted from a longer, more comprehensive questionnaire in *Learned Optimism* by Martin E. P. Seligman, Ph.D., vividly imagine yourself in each of the situations described, and choose one explanation. If neither cause seems to fit, choose one anyway. Don't choose the one you believe you should or the one that would seem right to other people. Be yourself, and decide which explanation is more likely to apply to you.

1. You forget your spouse's birthday.
_____ a. I'm not good at remembering birthdays.
_____ b. I was preoccupied with other things.

2. You owe the library a hefty fine for an overdue book.
_____ a. When I am really involved in what I am reading, I often forget when it's due.
_____ b. I was so involved in writing the report that I forgot to return the book.

3. You are penalized for not returning your income-tax forms on time.
_____ a. I always put off doing my taxes.
_____ b. I was lazy about getting my taxes done this year.

*continued*

4. You've been feeling run-down lately.
____ a. I never get a chance to relax.
____ b. I was exceptionally busy this week.

5. You lose your temper with a friend.
____ a. He/she is always nagging me.
____ b. He/she was in a hostile mood.

6. A friend says something that hurts your feelings.
____ a. My friend always blurts things out without thinking of others.
____ b. My friend was in a bad mood and took it out on me.

7. You fall down a great deal while skiing.
____ a. Skiing is difficult.
____ b. The trails were icy that day.

8. You gain weight over the holidays, and you can't lose an ounce.
____ a. Diets don't work in the long run.
____ b. The diet I tried didn't work.

**Total:** _____

## INTERPRETING YOUR ANSWERS

Give yourself 1 point for every (a.) answer, 0 for every (b.) answer. The lower your total score, the more optimistic you are. A total of 0 or 1 means you are extremely optimistic, 3 or 4 equates to about average in optimism, and anything higher means you're a pessimist!

# 58

# RETIREMENT PLANNING

### Rustproof Those Later Years

**Retirement** is generally viewed as a time of intellectual rustiness, life relegated to the mental slow lane. But it doesn't have to be that way.

You can have the same intellectual sharpness and zest for living at 75 that you have at 55 or even younger, if you put your mind to it—and start today. Here's how the experts say people in their preretirement years can prep their mental machinery for years and years of rust-free action.

#### EMBRACE MENTAL AND PHYSICAL CHALLENGES

"The adage 'use it or lose it' applies to the mind as well as the muscles," says Marian Diamond, Ph.D., a professor of neurosciences at the University of California, Berkeley. Just as muscles grow with physical exercise, the nerve cells in the brain expand with mental challenges.

Nerve cells have branches called dendrites that act like miniature telephone lines, allowing the cells to communicate with each other. Research shows that the brain cells of animals housed in intellectually enriched environments—with stimulating toys and the company of other animals—have more of these dendrites than the brain cells of animals kept in toyless solitude.

"The same goes for humans," says Dr. Diamond. "Studies

show that the area in the brain devoted to word understanding is significantly larger in the average college graduate than in the average high school graduate. Why? Because college graduates spend more time working with words."

**Challenge yourself.** Dr. Diamond urges people in their mid-career years to challenge themselves intellectually every day with anything from crossword puzzles to learning new languages to a new job. "At age 64," she says, "I became the director of the Lawrence Hall of Science at Berkeley, which designs science and math curricula for the nation's elementary schools. I wanted the stimulation and challenge, and I couldn't think of a better way to keep my mind from getting rusty than to devote myself to getting children interested in and excited about math and science."

**But don't overdo it.** Just be careful not to provide *too much* mental stimulation. When the toys used to enrich experimental animal environments are changed too often, the animals' brains do not develop as much as those with less stimulation, Dr. Diamond says. "Too much stimulation loses its value. By all means, enrich your mental life, but allow yourself adequate time to assimilate new information.

**Harness the mental power of exercise.** While your brain needs mental stimulation to stay sharp, a growing body of evidence shows that it needs *exercise* as well. According to a study by Robert Dustman, Ph.D., a research psychologist at the Salt Lake City Veterans Administration Medical Center, a little aerobic exercise can improve short-term memory, creativity and reaction time.

And that's not all. Other research points to the strong possibility that regular workouts may sharpen your sense of taste, stave off depression and enhance your reasoning abilities. The best part of these studies is that they weren't conducted on a bunch of cleat-shod youngsters. The razor-sharp folks who were tested ranged from 55 to 91.

## DEVELOP INTERESTS, OLD AND NEW

Difficult as this may seem, carve out some time—even a few hours a week—when you can step back from your daily responsibilities and indulge in some nonwork activity you truly enjoy. This doesn't mean heading for the hammock with a back scratcher and a beer. It means getting involved with a hobby—especially one that has the potential of becoming more than just a pastime.

"Hobbies are enriching at any age," says 65-year-old Ron Lawrence, M.D., neurologist at the University of California, Los Angeles, School of Medicine. "But they become crucial as retirement looms because they enhance self-esteem and confer a sense of identity at a time when your work identity may be disappearing."

Dr. Lawrence enjoys several hobbies: photography, painting, astronomy and ham radio. He says the best time to get serious about hobbies is during the mid-career years, when you generally feel sure of your interests and usually have some money to spend on them.

Hobbies also present brain-preserving mental challenges and opportunities to make new friends. And the sense of accomplishment that comes from mastering anything from baking to woodworking helps offset the loss of career accomplishments during retirement.

"Hobbies and social involvement are especially important to type-A men," says psychologist Allen Elkin, Ph.D., director of the Stress Management and Counseling Center in New York. "A client of mine retired a very rich man at the age of 50 but quickly became depressed because he had lost his job identity. Type A's can't simply lie on a beach. Anyone who derives most of their identity from their profession is going to need other sources of self-esteem to fall back on when they leave that profession behind."

Volunteering—whether to lead a scout troop or help out at an animal shelter—can also give meaning to your life and help you maintain ties to the community when retired.

## CHERISH PEOPLE AROUND YOU

Close ties to family and friends do a great deal more than make your life—both now and after retirement—more fulfilling. Social support just might extend your life. In a classic experiment, researchers at the University of California, Berkeley, asked several thousand residents of Alameda County,

California, to complete an extensive lifestyle questionnaire. After about ten years, they compared the answers of those who had died with those still living. Those who had died tended to be considerably more socially isolated than those who'd survived. Here's what you can do to keep relationships—and maybe yourself—alive.

**Make time for each other.** "The average mid-career couple spends only about 10 minutes a day talking to each other," Dr. Elkin says. "Retirement greatly expands that time, and problems can develop if spouses don't have activities they can enjoy together." Use vacations as retirement test runs. You've got money to spend, time to kill and the chance to devote more than 10 or 15 uninterrupted minutes to your spouse.

**Start exploring joint activities.** That way you'll not only find out what tickles your co-fancy, you'll also pick up just enough expertise to become truly excited at the prospect of the extra time retirement will provide to hone your skills. Maybe it's skiing, golf or ballroom dancing—even building a house. The possibilities are limitless. But one thing is for sure: Mutual interests help keep you mutually interested in each other.

**Make new friends.** As the years pass, it often seems harder and harder to make new friends. Part of the problem is that people tend to feel constrained by family and career responsibilities. They have much less time to "hang out" than they used to. But equally important, after 55, people often fall into emotional ruts and stop reaching out to others whom they might find intellectually stimulating.

"One of the great things about hobbies, classes and organizations is that they introduce you to people who share your interests," Dr. Elkin says. "Those new friends not only make your shared activity more enjoyable, they also expand your personal network. You can meet their friends, and some of them might become your friends as well."

**But keep the old.** You might be the most mentally alive, intellectually supercharged person on earth, but that can be cold comfort if you feel alone, isolated and depressed. When was the last time you contacted your best friend in high school? Your college roommate? Favorite cousin? Army buddy? Or that valued co-worker who moved away?

"Some letting go is inevitable and healthy," says Dr. Elkin, "but old friends provide valuable emotional grounding. Their perspectives on your past can help you solve problems in the present and plan for the future. And their evolving interests can introduce you to stimulating new activities and new people you might enjoy." Keeping in touch also gives you more people and places to visit—now and after you retire.

## SCOUT OUT YOUR RETIREMENT HOME

The fact that vacation and retirement bear such a resemblance can be turned to your advantage. Why not use your next few vacations to scout out new terrain and find your potential retirement paradise?

"I love to travel," says retirement specialist L. Malcolm Rodman, "but I noticed that after a certain point in my life, I stopped viewing destinations as just exotic places to visit and started to seriously consider them as possible places to live when I retire." If you're going to do a bit of scouting, you may want to keep a few of Rodman's guidelines in mind.

**Visit in the off-season.** If the area is a tourist attraction, you'll want to see it when things *aren't* hustling and bustling. "Try Florida in the summer or Maine in the winter, and see if you still like the area when it's unpopular with the rest of the world," says Rodman.

**Ask around.** Ask local residents what they think are the most problematic challenges of the area. You may find that the Arizona heat isn't half as bad as the sandstorms that'll rip your skin.

**Check your checklist.** Make a recreational checklist and see if the area meets your needs. Green Mountain Falls, Colorado, may be wonderful for hiking, but the closest thing you'll find to a symphony orchestra may be a group of banjo players.

**Look for like-minded people.** Does the community have a house of worship that suits you? Are you a sensitive, artistic sort about to move to an area hours away from a museum? If you have nothing in common with the people around you, the risk of isolation is high.

**Survey medical-care facilities.** Does the community offer adequate medical services? Most places do these days. But if you're dreaming of a cabin in the northwestern corner of Montana, you may want to consider just how far away help may be in case of an emergency.

A change of locale alone won't necessarily rustproof your retirement. But add a pinch of mental stimulation, a dash of exercise, a teaspoon of camaraderie and a whole lot of fun with a spouse, and you'll have just the kind of polish you need to keep your mind, and your outlook, shiny and new for many years to come.

# 59

# STRESS

## Tension Tamers to Rely On

**Let's** face it: Sometimes, *every* day is a bad day. Cars break down. Relationships founder. Bosses rile you. Bills pile up on you. Stocks fall. Babies bawl. Things start to wear on you.

Virtually every organ in the body can be negatively affected by stress. Put too much stress on your body or mind, and you begin to suffer the consequences: fatigue, tension, anxiety, even physical illness. When you're under stress, the body releases chemicals that help meet the challenge at hand but can be harmful when pumped out unceasingly.

"The more a person is stressed, the more likely that individual will experience illness, particularly heart disease," says Nancy Frasure-Smith, Ph.D., who conducted a study of the effects of stress reduction on heart-disease patients in Montreal. But the good news is, you can do something about excessive stress. In Dr. Frasure-Smith's study, patients who were monitored for stress and given tips on reducing stress were only half as likely to die from cardiac problems as patients who did not get such help. Even a little effort in stress reduction can turn the tide: Only about six hours of nursing contact, which included reassurance, calming fears, answering questions and the like, made the difference between life and death.

Even better news: Research seems to suggest that the older we get, the better we handle stress. Mid-life can be a period of accelerated growth, renewal and fulfillment. "This makes tremendous sense," says Margaret Gatz, Ph.D., a psychologist at the University of Southern California in Los Angeles. "In mid-life, you are getting good at handling difficult situations that used to really throw you when you were younger."

## Relax, You Can Handle It

The best news of all: Although stress is serious business, you can control it without elaborate, expensive medical care. "Stress reduction may not have to be based on intervention by a healthcare professional," explains Dr. Frasure-Smith. Try these do-it-yourself strategies to relive the symptoms of stress. They're all practical, low- or no-cost measures. Best of all, they work.

**Soak your troubles away.** Take a warm bath and let stress go down the drain. "It's my daily oasis," says one working mother. "I get in that tub, and my troubles melt." It may sound like poetry, but the method has some science behind it. Warm baths work by relaxing the muscles but also perhaps by slightly heating the brain, which can be calming, say experts. Notice, the operative word for the water is *warm*. If it's too hot, it can shock the system and cause muscles to constrict. Water between 100° and 102° F (that's comfortably warm to the touch) is best. Soak for no more than 15 minutes. (People with diabetes in particular should avoid hot soaks.)

**Laugh at stress.** Humor is one of the best on-the-spot stress busters around. It's virtually impossible to feel bad in the middle of a belly laugh. If you're caught in a situation you can't escape from or change, humor may be the healthiest form of release from temporary stress.

A good laugh works against stress physiologically, too. After a slight rise in heart rate and blood pressure during the laugh itself, there's an immediate release: Muscles relax, and blood pressure sinks below pre-laugh levels. The brain may also emit endorphins, the same stress reducers that are triggered by exercise. A hearty ha-ha-ha even produces a temporary boost in levels of immunoglobulin A, a virus fighter.

**Adopt a dog, cat or goldfish.** Pets can be great stress reducers. For some people, their pet is like a psychiatrist they don't have to pay. Research has shown that heart-attack victims who have pets live longer, that pets can help ease household tensions and that simply watching tropical fish swimming lazily in a tank may lower blood pressure, at least temporarily. Also, pets can help bring out our lighter, more playful side.

**Say a prayer.** Prayer can be an effective way to evoke the stress-relieving relaxation response. Herbert Benson, M.D., associate professor of medicine at Harvard Medical School, taught patients this simple relaxation method: Make yourself comfortable, sit quietly, and silently repeat a word or phrase. "Eighty percent of my patients chose a word or prayer arising from their faith, even though they were offered the choice of other soothing words, such as *peace* or *ocean*," says Dr. Benson. And those people who used words related to their religion stayed with the program longer and enjoyed better results in terms of improved health.

**Strike up the band!** Maybe it's the rhythm, maybe the melody—whatever it is, music helps relieve tension and stress. Scientific studies show that music played for patients before, during or after surgery seems to reduce anxiety, lessen pain and speed recovery. When the music was played in the operating room, the patients required 50 percent less sedative!

Find your own comfort tones. If rock and roll helps you relax more than classical or New Age music, listen to rock.

**Picture a tranquil scene.** A mountain lake shimmers in the moonlight. . . . A meadow glistens at dawn. . . . A tranquil scene can help you become the picture of tranquillity. Though science has no explanation for this mysterious effect, in recent years evidence has accumulated that suggests the calming, tranquilizing power of attractive scenes. One study revealed that hospital patients whose rooms looked out on an area of trees recovered faster than those whose view was of a brick wall. A photograph can work, too, if you can enjoy the serenity of the setting just as you would if you were there.

**Stroll away from stress.** Walking helps dissipate harmful stress chemicals—instantly. You can also take a walk to avoid stressful situations or to clear your mind before facing pressure cookers you can't avoid. You can take a walking break at work to escape boring routine and reinvigorate yourself. Researchers tell us that a brisk walk can give you more energy than a sugary snack. It also helps to condition you so that stressful events take less of a toll.

**Exhale and say "Ahhh . . ."** "Deep breathing is one of

the simplest, yet most effective, stress-management techniques there is," says Dean Ornish, M.D., director of the Preventive Medicine Research Institute in Sausalito, California, and author of *Dr. Dean Ornish's Program for Reversing Heart Disease*. It works its magic by infusing the blood with extra oxygen and causing the body to release endorphins, the natural tranquilizing hormones.

To maximize the effect, slowly inhale through your nose, expanding your abdomen before allowing air to fill your chest. Slowly reverse the process when you exhale. Take a few minutes each day to practice this technique.

**Steer into a mental rest stop.** Allow your mind to become fixed on an intriguing sight, sound or smell. It can be a bird hopping around on a branch outside your window. It can be clouds floating by, the aroma of a freshly baked apple pie, people marching along the sidewalk, buildings reflecting the sunlight, a loved one's breathing. Don't try to make sense of your mental image. The idea is to take a breath of mental fresh air, to allow your mind to be free of judging and decision making for a few moments. Don't think about what happened yesterday or what might happen tomorrow. Simply allow your mind to shift briefly into neutral. Several of these mental rest stops throughout the day can add up to true relaxation.

Think of these as mini-meditations—or mindfulness meditations, as Jon Kabat-Zinn, Ph.D., director of the stress-reduction clinic at the University of Massachusetts Medical Center in Worcester, calls them. "You could define mindfulness as moment-to-moment awareness," explains Dr. Kabat-Zinn. "You start seeing that your mind is often stormy and agitated. By practicing mindfulness, you learn to live in and enjoy each moment and to be more balanced in the face of stress."

## PUT A LID ON STRESS EARLY ON

What's even better than dealing with stress? Preventing it in the first place. Consider these tips to keep stress from overwhelming your life.

**If you need help, *ask*.** Learning to share the load gets at the heart of stress. "Stress for many of us is a self-inflicted burlen," says psychologist Steven Fahrion, Ph.D., of the Menninger Clinic in Topeka, Kansas. Let others pitch in where they can and should. The idea is to delegate what you can so that you're able to spend more time on the things you must do.

**Make time to play.** Play for the fun of it. "A person in midlife transition can be addicted to work and feel guilty about playing," says Neil Fiore, Ph.D., a psychologist in Berkeley, California. "If he isn't producing, he feels he is doing nothing. In fact, studies have shown that peak performers take more than the average number of holidays—at least six weeks a year."

Dr. Fiore suggests you keep an "unschedule," a calendar on which you schedule only play—walks in the park, tennis games, time to goof off. Then fill in your work schedule around the good times.

**Build intimate bonds.** Learn to open up to others, to share your deepest feelings and to instill in others the trust to do the same. Psychologists tell us that intimacy is not only an immediate stress reducer, it also provides the kind of loving, nonjudgmental support that helps us develop confidence to deal with whatever life sends our way.

---

### ANTI-AGING CHECKUP
## 25 COMMON SIGNS AND SYMPTOMS OF STRESS

Here are common signs of stress, compiled by Paul J. Rosch, M.D., president of the American Institute of Stress in Yonkers, a nonprofit educational clearinghouse for information on stress. Check off the indicators below that fit your experience.

\_\_\_\_ Frequent headaches, jaw clenching or teeth grinding
\_\_\_\_ Neck ache, back pain or muscle spasms
\_\_\_\_ Frequent colds, infections or herpes sores
\_\_\_\_ Rashes, itching, hives or unexplained allergy attacks
\_\_\_\_ Difficulty breathing or frequent sighing
\_\_\_\_ Sudden attacks of panic

*continued*

_____ Chest pain, palpitations or rapid pulse
_____ Diminished sexual desire or performance
_____ Excess anxiety, worry, guilt or nervousness
_____ Increased anger, frustration or hostility
_____ Depression or frequent or wild mood swings
_____ Insomnia or nightmares
_____ Difficulty concentrating, forgetfulness, disorganization or confusion
_____ Trouble with making decisions
_____ Feeling overloaded or overwhelmed
_____ Sense of loneliness or worthlessness
_____ Nervous habits, such as fidgeting or foot tapping
_____ More frustration, irritability, edginess, defensiveness or suspiciousness than usual
_____ Increased number of minor accidents
_____ Reduced work efficiency or productivity
_____ Social withdrawal and isolation
_____ Constant tiredness, weakness or fatigue
_____ Significant weight gain or loss without diet change
_____ Increased smoking, alcohol, prescription or over-the counter drug use
_____ Lack of interest in appearance and punctuality

## INTERPRETING YOUR ANSWERS

More than a few check marks could signal stress overload. To determine whether these complaints are caused by stress or other problems, check with your physician.

# 60

# THINKING

How to Stay Smart for Life

**You've** probably heard the old saying "the mind is the first thing to go." But our ability to think clearly and solve problems doesn't have to deteriorate as a natural consequence of aging, says Eugene Raudsepp, Ph.D., president of Princeton Creative Research and author of *Creative Growth Games* and other books about mental skills.

"You can keep the brain very alive and active late in life," says Dr. Raudsepp. "I have always noticed that the older people in my seminars are better students. They are more serious and more motivated, and they spend more time and get more benefit from the homework."

And research supports Dr. Raudsepp's classroom experiences. When researchers at the University of Utah in Salt Lake City tested verbal analogical reasoning in people ranging in age from 20 to 79, they found that learning was *not* impaired in the older folks. Although the 60- and 70-year-olds tended to take a bit longer than younger test subjects, they did not make more mistakes.

## FIT BODY, FITTER BRAIN

So the sword of your wit may slow down a bit with age, but it need not grow dull. Practice these tips to help you keep it razor sharp.

**Aim for good health.** Much of the deterioration of mental abilities that was once believed to be a natural consequence of aging is actually a result of illness. "In the presence of good health, mental functioning remains very much intact," says Gene Cohen, M.D., Ph.D., director of the Washington, D.C., Center on Aging, and former acting director of the National Institute on Aging (NIA), part of the National Institutes of Health in Bethesda, Maryland.

One of the most recently discovered causes of mental deterioration is high blood pressure. An NIA-sponsored study found that men who had had high blood pressure for more than ten years had significant deadening of left-brain tissue and major increases in fluid on both sides of their brains—an indication of actual loss of brain tissue. "This damage, in time, may express itself in problems with memory, language and finding your way around," says Declan Murphy, M.D., senior staff fellow at the laboratory of neurosciences at NIA. "If you can prevent high blood pressure from occurring with diet and exercise—and then maintain that state—you may be able to prevent these brain abnormalities from occurring."

**Under pressure? Take a walk.** A regular program of aerobic exercise—such as walking, running or swimming for 20 minutes, three times a week—can apparently maintain and even boost your ability to think and react quickly. In a study reported in the *Research Quarterly for Exercise and Sport*, reaction time improved significantly in a group of women one year after they took up a program of exercise three times a week.

"These people were able to improve their ability to think fast under pressure," says Roberta E. Rikli, Ph.D., a professor in the department of health, physical education and recreation at California State University, Fullerton. "Exercise helps increase the production of brain chemicals that are vital for processing information. More important, it helps boost oxygen and blood flow to the brain, which improves function." Exercise may also affect brain structure by causing improvements in nerve passageways.

**Cheer up.** You may never have thought that being down in the dumps can affect how you *think*, but it apparently can. When researchers studied 72 elderly people at the University of North Texas in Denton, they found that those who were depressed had more difficulty than nondepressed people when it came to solving tiring tasks that involved short-term memory.

**Sniff for success.** Scientists believe that certain scents can improve mental alertness and performance. Studies at the University of Cincinnati and at Catholic University of America in Washington, D.C., found that the aromas of peppermint and lily of the valley boosted the mental performance of test subjects.

And in Japan, researchers found that when keyboard operators got a whiff of lemon-scented air, their errors dropped 54 percent. A jasmine fragrance resulted in a 33 percent drop in errors, and lavender was linked with a 21 percent drop. The smells appear to directly stimulate the brain, though researchers don't know exactly how. But it couldn't hurt to try scenting your work area with flowers or lemon.

### BE A RATIONAL THINKER

Once you've set the stage for successful, clear thinking, here's how to go about it.

**Get the facts, ma'am.** Not just the obvious ones, but everything you can get your hands on. "Mistakes are usually made because someone has insufficient or bad data," says John C. Johnson, M.D., director of emergency medical services at Porter Memorial Hospital in Valparaiso, Indiana.

"We tend to have a lot of fixed ideas that are not too creative," says Dr. Raudsepp. "When you brainstorm, initially you get ideas that 98 percent of people have. But if you continue to generate ideas and alternatives, more effective and original ideas will emerge."

**Look at the other side.** To be a cool thinker and prevent being lured into making bad decisions, view things with a critical eye. There's no better way to find holes in faulty thinking than to ask yourself, "What are the reasons I may be wrong?" When time allows, consult with another person, preferably someone who thinks differently than you.

**Examine your real needs.** The key to rational thinking and clear decision making is to remain flexible. Listen to your inner self. Do you hear a cranky little voice inside saying "I must have this. . . . I must . . . I must . . . I must!"? Many people have the tendency to take their important desires and turn them into "musts." So the next time you hear yourself saying "I must," step back and ask yourself, "Must I?"

---

**ANTI-AGING CHECKUP**
# HOW EASILY DISTRACTED ARE YOU?

This test was developed by Stanley Coren, Ph.D., professor of psychology at the University of British Columbia in Vancouver, and used in his research on distractibility. "The test measures arousability: People who are highly arousable are also highly distractible," says Dr. Coren. "The higher your score, the more likely you are to be distracted. The more distractible you are, the more difficult you may find it to concentrate and think clearly."

To measure your distractibility, answer each of the following questions with either: Never (or Almost Never), Seldom, Occasionally, Frequently or Always (or Almost Always).

_____ 1. I am a calm person.

_____ 2. I get flustered if I have several things to do.

_____ 3. Sudden changes of any kind produce an immediate emotional effect on me.

_____ 4. Strong emotions carry over for one or two hours after I leave the situation that caused them.

_____ 5. I am restless and fidgety.

_____ 6. My mood is quickly influenced by entering new places.

_____ 7. I get excited easily.

_____ 8. I find that my heart keeps beating fast for a while after I have been "stirred up."

_____ 9. I can be emotionally moved by what other people consider to be simple things.

_____ 10. I startle easily.

_____ 11. I am easily frustrated.

_____ 12. I tend to remain excited or moved for a long period of time after seeing a good movie.

**Total:** _____

*continued*

**INTERPRETING YOUR ANSWERS**

For question 1, give yourself 5 points for Never, 4 for seldom, 3 for Occasionally, 2 for Frequently and 1 for Always. For questions 2 through 12, give yourself 1 point for each Never, 2 for Seldom, 3 for Occasionally, 4 for Frequently and 5 for Always.

Add up your total score. For women, a score of 41 or above puts you in the top 25 percent of people who are most distractible. For men, a score of 37 or above will put you in the "highly distractible" range.

### PAY ATTENTION!

Your ability to think clearly and effectively may have nothing to do with your age or your intelligence. It may hinge on how easily distracted you are, says Stanley Coren, Ph.D., professor of psychology at the University of British Columbia in Vancouver and coauthor of *Prediction of Physiological Arousability*. Dr. Coren's research has found that people react differently to noises, interruptions and mental distractions.

If you know you are distractible (you can find out by completing the "Anti-Aging Checkup" on page 356), Dr. Coren recommends the following strategies.

**Block out distractions.** "Do your thinking in a quiet, less distracting place," suggests Dr. Coren. Reduce other distractions as much as possible. For example, turn off the television and telephone, find a quiet room decorated in peaceful colors, and close the door.

**Build patterns.** "Develop a set of habits so that you always work at the same place at roughly the same time," says Dr. Coren. "Have a special table or desk at which you do only your problem solving or thinking or other work. Schedule a special time for that work, and stick to it on a regular basis.

"The reason is, we often get distracted by the very problem of making the decisions as to where to work, when to work, how to prepare the area for work and so on. If you set up reliable patterns, these decisions are made automatically, and you're not distracted by the little details," says Dr. Coren.

**Scribble down your thoughts.** "Carry a little notebook and write things down," says Dr. Coren. "The motto is 'The faintest ink is better than the strongest memory.'" Jotting down key points in your thought processes can also help you find your way back to significant ideas at a later time. Don't depend on your memory to hold on to everything.

**Keep your cool.** "If you are distractible, do what you can, but don't worry about it. If you worry about being distracted, that in itself is a distraction," says Dr. Coren. "Some people get so worried about forgetting that they forget what they were trying to think about."

# 61

# WORRY

### Free Yourself from Fretting

**Sometimes** it's tough not to anguish about things that have happened. You keep saying to yourself, "If only I hadn't lost my temper" or "I really should have taken that other job."

Or maybe you fret about things that *could* happen: Your dinner party might be a flop. You might lose your job. You may become ill. Your house might burn down.

Why let these unsettling thoughts intrude into our minds? "You don't really *want* to keep worrying, but you think you can't help it," says Paula Levine, Ph.D., director of the Agoraphobia Resource Center in Coral Gables, Florida.

And some worriers think their worrying *helps*. "Some people believe that their worrying keeps awful things from happening," explains Dr. Levine. "It gives them a feeling of being in control. They really think that if they were to stop worrying, awful things would happen. The worrying feels active, feels powerful, feels like they're doing something about it."

But worrying can cause enormous amounts of stress. Not only can you lose sleep, but when the "what if?" and "if only" thoughts take over, they can sap your energy and enthusiasm.

#### KEEP WORRY AT BAY

Think it's time to drive away those worrisome thoughts? Try out these tips.

**Take action.** Do something positive to remove the reason you worry. If you fear you'll oversleep and miss that important morning appointment, for example, set *two* alarm clocks, one electric and one windup in case the power goes out.

"Most people worry about their house being robbed," says Dr. Levine. "But you can do something about it. You can make sure you have appropriate locks, you can install an alarm, you can take special precautions. You can even move to a safer neighborhood."

**Envision success.** Researchers at Washington State University in Pullman found that visualization significantly lowered apprehension associated with public speaking. The subjects pictured the best possible scenario for the day of their speech: putting on the right clothes, feeling clear, confident and thoroughly prepared and giving a smooth, brilliant talk.

"You can use this to prepare for any task, be it public speaking, a sports competition or a project at work," says Theodore S. Hopf, Ph.D., associate professor of communications at Washington State University. First, imagine your task as a positive experience. Use as much detail as possible. Write down a scenario to establish it in your mind. Then relax, breathe deeply and read the scenario to yourself. Do this several times before the date of your task.

**Hit the road.** Physical exercise of any kind can help defuse anxiety. "A lot of worry will be fueled by the fact that you're tense," says Daniel S. Wegner, Ph.D., professor of psychology at the University of Virginia in Charlottesville. "A good workout will drain some of that. Any exercise that tends to de-stress you would be good."

Studies at the University of Wisconsin-Madison, for example, found that people who were worried, frustrated or fearful scored much lower on anxiety tests after they went for a run.

**List reasons not to worry.** Can't get worries about your upcoming vacation out of your mind? Try making a list of reasons the trip won't be a disaster. If you're worried about missing your plane, for instance, list the reasons you *won't:* You've checked your reservation time, you've arranged for transportation, you've allowed an extra hour at the airport. A study at the Medical Research Council Applied Psychology Unit in Cambridge, England, revealed that people worry about things that might happen because they're not as good at thinking about why something *won't* happen. When worriers listed reasons the event wasn't likely to take place, anxiety was reduced and worry levels decreased.

## DEFUSE UNREASONABLE WORRY

You can't run away from, ignore or overpower your worries. The harder you try, the stronger they'll get. "When you have a worry or a fear, it's something you're afraid to confront and deal with directly. So you try to avoid it," says Dr. Wegner. "But the thought comes back as an intrusive thought rather than as something you're thinking about on purpose. And then it's more alarming because the thought 'happens' to you at inappropriate times. When you try not to think about something, it comes back with a vengeance. It surprises you and can create a very strong emotional reaction."

The solution? Confront your worries. Here's how.

**Limit your worries to one hour.** If you spend an hour a day actively worrying about your problems—you'll have 23 worry-free hours a day! And by confronting your worst worries, you can help defuse your anxiety.

"Many people believe that if they actively tried to concentrate on their worries, the worries would somehow overwhelm them. That's not going to happen," says Dr. Wegner. "In fact, if you actively try to think about what's worrying you, you'll actually reduce your sensitivity to it, compared with when you're trying to ignore it. People usually find that thinking about it on purpose is easier and not nearly as anxiety-producing. You grow accustomed to the thought, so the emotion-producing quality of the thought decreases."

**Try a worry chair.** Dr. Levine uses a similar strategy with worriers. "I tell the worriers to organize all the worrying into one special time and one special place. I call that the worry chair. I tell them to pick a time when nobody else is home, when you're not going to be interrupted. If the phone rings, don't answer it. If you're afraid you might not worry long enough, set the alarm clock. I don't want you to stop until it goes off.

"They come in a week or two later and say, 'I couldn't do it for an hour.' So I tell them to try it for 45 minutes. Before too long, they've reduced their worrying to a very short time."

**Distract yourself.** What do you do until your "worry hour" arrives? Consciously direct your mind to think about something else that can absorb your thoughts: your work, the movie you saw last night, an upcoming vacation or party. "This is a short-term strategy," cautions Dr. Wegner. "You're going to have to deal with the worry at some point. But the idea is that you may be better able to deal with it later, when it's not getting in the way of your daily activities."

**Find a friendly ear.** You may be able to vent your worry by talking to a friend or a therapist. "Talking about it can help free you from being obsessed with the worry—kind of like taking the cork out of the bottle," says Dr. Wegner. "Sometimes a good friend can do it. But a lot of times, friends want us to be happy, so friends may simply try to help us avoid the problem."

You may need the help of a therapist, who can help guide you to think about your worst fears and deal with your most troublesome thoughts. "In doing that, the person gets over the avoidance and suppression that has made the thoughts so special and so powerful," explains Dr. Wegner.

---

### ANTI-AGING CHECKUP
## ARE YOU A WORRYWART?

Are your worries reasonable or unfounded? To help you find out, answer the following questions Yes or No.

_____ 1. Do you feel that you must worry before major events in your life?

_____ 2. Does it take you more than ten minutes to fall asleep at night?

_____ 3. Do you find yourself distracted by worry even during enjoyable moments, such as while reading a book, watching a movie or making love?

_____ 4. Do you worry about things you have no control over?

_____ 5. If you've done everything you possibly can about a certain situation or event, do you still worry about it?

_____ 6. If something goes well, do you worry about what "might have happened"?

*continued*

_____ 7. Do you ever worry about something so much that you don't do it, like going to a party, taking a trip or going to the store?

_____ 8. Do you always find something to worry about, even when life is really okay?

_____ 9. Do you have great difficulty turning off your worries?

_____ 10. Does your worry ever lead to uncomfortable physical symptoms, such as shortness of breath, racing heartbeat, sweaty palms, weakness in the arms and legs, blurred vision or butterflies in the stomach?

**Total:** _____

## INTERPRETING YOUR ANSWERS

Give yourself 1 point for every Yes. If your score is 0 to 1, you're basically worry-free. If your score is 2 to 3, you're a mild worrier.

If you scored 4 or more, of if you answered Yes to question 7 or 10, then you are definitely a worrywart. "If you score that high, you should seriously think about seeing a therapist because it sounds like your worrying is interfering with your life," says Paula Levine, Ph.D., director of the Agoraphobia Resource Center in Coral Gables, Florida.

# ABOUT THE AUTHOR

Tom Monte is a medical journalist, former editor of *Nutrition Action*, a publication of the Center for Science in the Public Interest, and former associate editor of *East West Journal*. His work has appeared in the *Chicago Tribune, Runner's World, Life* and *The Saturday Evening Post*, among others.

Tom's previous books include *Pritikin: The Man Who Healed America's Heart* (Rodale Press, 1988) and *World Medicine: East West Guide to Healing Your Body* (Jeremy P. Tarcher, 1993). Tom also coauthored *Recalled by Life: The Story of My Recovery from Cancer* with Anthony Sattilaro, M.D. (Houghton Mifflin, 1982), a best-seller in the United States and abroad.

Tom lives in Amherst, Massachusetts, with his wife and three children.

# INDEX

Note: <u>Underscored</u> page references indicate boxed text. Brand names of prescription medications are denoted by the symbol Rx.